Welcome to the EVERYTHING® seies!

These handy, accessible books give you all you need to tackle a difficult project, gain a new hobby, comprehend a fascinating topic, prepare for an exam, or even brush up on something you learned back in school but have since forgotten.

You can read an *EVERYTHING®* book from cover-to-cover or just pick out the information you want from our four useful boxes: e-facts, e-ssentials, e-alerts, and e-questions. We literally give you everything you need to know on the subject, but throw in a lot of fun stuff along the way, too.

We now have well over 100 *EVERYTHING®* books in print, spanning such wide-ranging topics as weddings, pregnancy, wine, learning guitar, one-pot cooking, managing people, and so much more. When you're done reading them all, you can finally say you know *EVERYTHING®*!

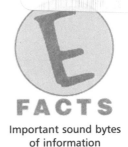

FACTS

Important sound bytes
of information

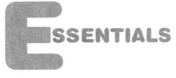

SSENTIALS

Quick handy tips

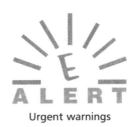

ALERT

Urgent warnings

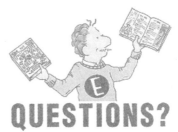

QUESTIONS?

Solutions to
common problems

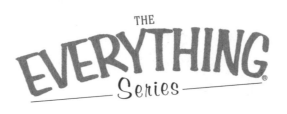

THE
EVERYTHING®
Series

Dear Reader:

If you're like me, you're not looking forward to getting older. But what can you do about it? Well, plenty, actually. And that's what this book is all about—inexpensive and effective ways to slow the aging process so that you get the maximum enjoyment out of life.

As I researched and wrote *The Everything® Anti-aging Book,* I became painfully aware of how little I was doing to stay youthful and healthy. My diet was full of all of the wrong things (such as steak and hamburgers—two of my favorite foods!), I wasn't getting nearly enough exercise, and I wasn't taking advantage of the many useful age-slowing dietary supplements currently on the market.

But that's all changed. I now eat with nutrition in mind, walk every day (well, almost every day), and take saw palmetto and ginkgo biloba, among other supplements. Writing this book showed me the light, and I hope that reading it will do the same for you. I tried very hard to make anti-aging as fun and exciting as possible so that you will be entertained and motivated, as well as educated. And I believe that I've succeeded in achieving that goal.

In closing, let me remind you that slowing the aging process is as much mental as it is physical. If you think young, you'll stay young. So make sure you exercise your brain as well as your body!

Sincerely,

Donald Vaughan

THE
EVERYTHING®
ANTI-AGING
BOOK

Discover the secrets of
looking young, feeling great,
and having boundless energy

Donald Vaughan

Adams Media Corporation
Avon, Massachusetts

EDITORIAL
Publishing Director: Gary M. Krebs
Managing Editor: Kate McBride
Copy Chief: Laura MacLaughlin
Project Editor: Bethany Brown

PRODUCTION
Production Director: Susan Beale
Production Manager: Michelle Roy Kelly
Series Designer: Daria Perreault
Layout and Graphics: Arlene Apone,
Paul Beatrice, Brooke Camfield,
Colleen Cunningham, Daria Perreault,
Frank Rivera

An Everything® Series Book.
Everything® is a registered trademark of Adams Media Corporation.

Published by Adams Media Corporation
57 Littlefield Street, Avon, MA 02322
www.adamsmedia.com

ISBN: 1-58062-565-7
Printed in the United States of America.

J I H G F E D C B A

Library of Congress Cataloging-in-Publication Data
Vaughan, Donald.
The everything anti-aging book / by Donald Vaughan.
p.   cm.
Includes index.
ISBN 1-58062-565-7
1. Longevity. 2. Aging. 3. Health.
RA776.75 .V38 2001
613–dc21   201046322

Illustrations by Barry Littmann.

This book is available at quantity discounts for bulk purchases.
For information, call 1-800-872-5627.

Visit the entire Everything® series at everything.com

Contents

Acknowledgments

To my wife, Nanette, and my parents,
Donald and Shirley Vaughan, for their
unwavering love, support, and encouragement.

Introduction

Unfortunately for all of us, aging is an inevitable part of life. However, the thought of aging doesn't have to (and shouldn't) make us cringe. In fact, if we take a proactive approach toward developing an anti-aging regimen grounded in nutrition, exercise, and healthful living, we can embrace our later years as some of the best years of our lives. We don't have to wait for future science to slow the aging process—there's plenty we can do right now to hedge our bet against Father Time.

Nearly everything in our lives, from the food we eat, to the work we do, to the activities we enjoy on our days off, has an impact on how our bodies age. Some of these factors accelerate the aging process; others help slow it down. The one thing they all have in common is that we can influence them—for good or bad—if we choose to.

Indeed, how well we age and, ultimately, how long we live have as much, if not more, to do with the many lifestyle choices we make every day as with our genetic background, risk of chronic illness, or any number of other uncontrollable factors. Bottom line: It really is possible to age well if you're willing to work at it.

Throughout this book, we'll discuss the many lifestyle factors that affect the aging process and what we can do to maximize the good and minimize the bad. Make sure you share this information with your friends and loved ones; adding useful, healthful years to our lives is much easier when it's a group effort.

CHAPTER 1

Starting Out Right

Benjamin Franklin once noted that the only certainties in life are death and taxes. However, most doctors would probably agree that old Ben was wrong; a third certainty faces us all—and that is aging. Indeed, aging is an inescapable part of being alive. From the moment we're conceived until we reach our final resting place, the aging process slowly, perniciously affects our bodies and our minds. You can fight it—and many of us do—but you can't stop it.

The Quest for Immortality

For most of us, the so-called "ravages of time" don't really become apparent until we reach our thirtieth or fortieth birthdays. Only then, at the first sign of gray hair and wrinkles (the time-honored badges of middle age), does the realization that we're growing older really begin to sink in; only then do thoughts of our own mortality become increasingly common.

Most people, of course, consider themselves immortal for the first twenty years or so of their lives. Aging is what their parents do—not them. In one of life's more cruel jests, children can't wait to grow older, while older people wish that they were young again. Whoever said that youth is wasted on the young is absolutely right—in the eyes of almost everyone over fifty!

Without question, age plays a vital role in the development of disease. Though infection and a handful of childhood disorders are more common in young people, most degenerative diseases afflict people over forty. This includes Alzheimer's disease, most forms of cancer, osteoporosis, heart disease, non-insulin-dependent diabetes, stroke, and osteoarthritis. These and many other diseases are health-affecting bombs waiting to be triggered by advancing age—which is one of the most important reasons, perhaps, for researchers to strive so hard to better understand the aging process.

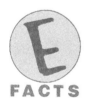

FACTS

In ancient Greece and Rome, elderly men were encouraged to sleep beside young virgins to reclaim their youthful vigor. The concept was based on the amazing longevity of a guy named Hermippus, who ran a school for young girls and who, supposedly, lived to be 150 years old.

Until very recently, of course, there wasn't much we could do to hold at bay the aging process. Doctors advised their patients to eat right and get more exercise, but they had very little else to offer in terms of helping their clients stay young and vibrant. For most physicians, old age was (and still is) more of a label than something to be studied and treated.

Over the past two decades, however, researchers around the world have made astounding advances in their understanding of how aging affects the body and what can be done to slow it down. For example, researchers know more now than ever before about the importance of proper nutrition in keeping the body healthy and young; replacement body parts are being successfully grown in the laboratory; and the international Human Genome Project promises to help eliminate or cure a wide variety of conditions that in the past cut life short at a tragically early age, or made growing older a painful burden. Prehistoric people were extraordinarily lucky if they lived to the ripe old age of twenty; however, children born today, researchers say, can expect to live well into their seventies, eighties, and beyond in relatively good health.

And what will the future hold? The prospects are simply unbelievable. Some futurists believe that if science continues its current pace, man will one day live 130, 140, even 150 healthful years. It may sound like science fiction now, but so did space travel just fifty years ago.

At the moment, 120 years is considered the absolute limit of human longevity. It's simply impossible, scientists say, for the human machine to function much longer than that, no matter how healthful our lifestyle. But in the minds of many age specialists, a 120-year lifespan is a barrier that can and will be broken, much like the 4-minute mile. Before Roger Bannister shattered that record on May 6, 1954, with a time of 3 minutes, 59.4 seconds, more than one doctor said it was a physical impossibility, that the human body—no matter how hard you trained—simply could not sustain the speed needed to run a mile in under 4 minutes. Yet Roger Bannister proved them wrong, and science may one day do the same in regard to human longevity.

Current and future breakthroughs in the science of aging promise to raise some intriguing moral and ethical questions. Even if we could live to be 150, would we want to? What quality of life could people that old expect? What burdens would they place on society in regard to health care, population, and so forth? What are the emotional and psychological implications of extreme longevity? And, of course, where do we draw the line? In theory, nutrition supplementation, gene therapy, laboratory organ growth/natural regeneration, and approaches that are now only in the conceptual stage could one day give us Immortal Man and Immortal Woman—humans capable of living not just decades but literally centuries. The prospect, while currently outside of the realm of possibility, gives us food for thought.

Our quest for immortality is far from a modern concern. Ever since early humans were first able to grasp the concepts of time and age, we've been trying desperately to find a way to stop the clock. Spanish explorer Juan Ponce de Leon became the first European to visit what is now the state of Florida as a result of his quest for the fabled Fountain of Youth, and many, many others have followed different paths in the hope of making similar dreams a reality.

We now know, of course, that there is no Fountain of Youth, no simple elixir or pill that will instantly erase the signs and symptoms of age. However, there are many easy and effective ways to slow the aging process and, in some situations, to actually reverse it. For example, many of us can greatly extend our life span simply by making a few important lifestyle changes, such as eating less red meat and more vegetables, exercising a few days a week, and not smoking.

It's vitally important that anti-aging not be approached in a haphazard manner, however. Simply "thinking young" when it's convenient will do little to add extra years to your life. To age well and stay as young as possible, it's necessary to formulate a comprehensive anti-aging regimen—a game plan, if you will—that improves every aspect of your physical and mental well-being on a day-to-day basis. Tips for such a regimen can be found throughout this book.

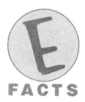

FACTS

In 1889, seventy-two-year-old Parisian neurologist Charles-Edouard Brown-Sequard announced that he had developed an anti-aging elixir derived from dog and guinea pig testicles. The good doctor injected himself with the concoction and announced that he never felt better. He died five years later.

It's also important that you work closely with your doctor in formulating and maintaining your anti-aging regimen. After all, no one knows more about your physical and mental health than your personal physician, and his or her input can go a long way toward creating the personalized game plan that most effectively addresses your specific needs and goals. Frequent consultation with your doctor is also valuable because he or she will be well versed in the pros and cons of the latest anti-aging technologies, supplements, and approaches.

Over the course of this book, we'll examine how and why the body ages, what factors influence our rate and degree of aging, and what we can do to stay as young as possible for as long as possible. Always remember, however: It's not the years in your life that really matter but the life in your years. No matter how long you live, life is still short. Enjoy it while you can.

Working with Your Doctor

Selecting the right doctor is one of the most important decisions you can make when it comes to your health and longevity. However, in this era of managed care and "here today, gone tomorrow" health programs, choosing the doctor who's best for you isn't as easy as it once was. It's important that you do your homework and ask a lot of questions before making your final decision.

Finding Common Ground

One of the most important considerations, of course, is how attuned your physician is to you, your needs, and your goals. In addition to your primary health care, it's essential that your doctor share your anti-aging philosophy, that he or she understand how important it is to you to live as many good years as you possibly can. Many so-called "old school" doctors aren't exactly advocates of the holistic approach to medicine and couldn't care less about your desire to incorporate health, nutrition, and breaking advances in science and medicine to help you live longer. These physicians—and fortunately there are fewer and fewer of them—prefer instead merely to treat your problem de jour and send you on your way.

Compatibility is essential in fostering a good relationship with your physician. It is hoped that you will be working very closely together not only in maintaining your health but also in designing the anti-aging regimen that is best for you. Your doctor should be well versed in the importance of nutrition, exercise, lifestyle, and science—today's and tomorrow's—in adding years to your life and life to your years. Ideally, the two of you will share responsibility for a common goal: helping you live as long as you possibly can. And this requires much more than a five-minute physical and yearly flu shot.

FACTS

The Internet is replacing doctor visits for a growing number of Americans. In fact, close to 70 million Americans have searched the Internet for health information. The top five illnesses that people research online include depression, allergies, cancer, bipolar disorder, and arthritis.

One would think that all doctors would share this vision, but such is not the case. Many doctors, especially those working for managed care companies, are lucky if they get to spend a full ten minutes with each patient. Under such stringent time constraints, it's all they can do to evaluate and treat whatever it is that brought you to their office that day, check your vitals, and usher you out. An extended discussion regarding the best anti-aging supplements for you simply doesn't figure into their schedule. This is the kind of doctor you want to avoid, if at all possible.

Know Your Needs

People who get their health care through a managed care plan may feel they are stuck with whichever doctor they first see, but this usually isn't the case. While there are restrictions, most managed care plans offer a selection of physicians from which to choose—and it's up to you to choose wisely. Before you pick up the phone, ask yourself the following:

- How important is the gender of your physician? Some people feel more comfortable with doctors who are the same gender as they are, while others don't care.
- How aggressively do you want your health treated? Some people are really gung ho where their health is concerned, while others prefer a more conservative approach. Your doctor should share the same philosophy, within reason.
- Would you feel more comfortable with an advanced practice nurse, such as a nurse practitioner or physician's assistant, as your primary

care provider? Studies have shown that advanced practice nurses are more holistic in their approach to health care and are usually able to spend more time with their patients.

Things to Consider

Communication is the key to success in choosing a qualified and understanding physician. When evaluating prospective physicians, consider the following questions:

- Will this doctor take the time to talk and listen to me, or is he or she in too much of a rush to see the next patient?
- Will this doctor answer my questions and provide me with sufficient information to make decisions?
- Will this doctor be willing to sit down and thoroughly discuss my concerns?
- Is this doctor available by telephone? How about by e-mail? (While you shouldn't expect any doctor to drop everything whenever you call, a good doctor will return your calls within an hour if it's an emergency, and within two days for general health questions.)
- Can I have faith and place my trust in him or her?

Other items to consider when choosing a doctor include his ability or willingness to do the following:

- Plan ahead to prevent problems.
- Review your total health program regularly.
- Prescribe medication carefully and only when needed.
- Emphasize preventative care and maintenance of good health. (This means helping you lose weight or stop smoking if you ask him to.)

Consider Your Options

If you are a member of a managed care plan, you were probably given a list of doctors in your area and asked to choose one as your primary care physician. But if you are not a member of a managed care

program or are new to an area, things can be a little more difficult. The one thing you should NOT do is select your doctor from the Yellow Pages. Instead, ask friends and relatives for recommendations or call the county or state medical society for a referral list. Avoid commercial hospital or physician referral services because they often have a bias toward members, some
of whom may have paid for the privilege of being listed.

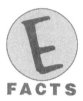

FACTS

Medicine that was once only science fiction may soon become science fact as researchers use genomics and stem-cell biology to perfect treatments that rely less on the use of a scalpel and more on the body's amazing ability to heal itself. Regenerative medicine will take medicine to a whole new level, researchers say, by making failing systems as good as new, rather than just patching them up.

Once you have narrowed your list, call to see whether the physician is accepting new patients and, if so, whether you can make an appointment for a brief patient interview. Some doctors will say yes, and some won't (often with the explanation that it takes valuable time away from other patients). If you do receive an appointment, expect to be charged. After all, time is money—especially to physicians. However, consider it money well spent if it helps you find the perfect doctor for you.

What to Ask

Questions to ask during your interview include the following:

- What are his or her office hours?
- Who is the on-call doctor when his or her office is closed?
- How long does it usually take to get an appointment for a routine visit?
- How much time is allowed for initial and routine visits?
- How are medical emergencies handled?
- Will the doctor discuss medical concerns over the phone?
- Does the doctor make house calls?
- Does the doctor have hospital privileges? If so, at which hospital?

- What are the office payment policies?
- What kinds of insurance does he or she accept?

Clearly describe your needs and expectations and ask to what degree you will be allowed to share in your medical decision making. Ideally, the relationship will be fifty-fifty; avoid a doctor who scorns patient input or seems to have a God complex. It's during your interview or, lacking that, your initial visit that you should bring up the issue of anti-aging and how important it is to you. Brownie points are scored if he embraces the topic and seems eager to help; avoid doctors who scoff at the notion or don't want to be bothered.

It's the Little Things That Matter

Here are some other considerations when selecting a doctor:

- Is the office located within a reasonable distance from your home?
- Was the doctor's office staff friendly, courteous, and helpful?
- Was the office clean and neat?
- How crowded was the waiting room? (A waiting room packed with patients could suggest that the doctor overbooks, causing everyone to wait.)
- Is the doctor board certified or board eligible? (Board certified means that he or she has two years or more of training in a specialty after graduation from medical school and has passed a national examination. Board eligible means that the training has been completed, but not the exam.)

Lifetime Checkups

Preventing illness means staying on top of your health through regular physical exams and checkups with your doctor. As each stage in life presents new medical challenges, knowing what to watch for as you continually grow older can be paramount to prevention and treatment. Let's go through a loose schedule of what you should keep an eye on through the various stages of your life.

Twenties and Thirties

You should be tested for HIV and hepatitis if you engage in risky sexual behavior (i.e., unprotected sex). Blood pressure should be checked at least every two years, skin every three years, and cholesterol every five years. You should also conduct a skin self-exam every month and receive a tetanus booster at least once every ten years. Women should receive a pelvic exam annually, a Pap test every one to two years, and a clinical breast exam every year, and they should perform a breast self-exam every month. Men should perform a testicular self-exam monthly.

Forties

Blood pressure should be tested at least every two years, cholesterol every five years, and skin every three years. You should also have an eye exam every three years. And you should receive a fasting plasma glucose test every three years after age forty-five. Women should receive a pelvic exam every year, a Pap test every one to two years, a mammogram every one to two years (depending on risk factors), and a clinical breast exam every year, and they should perform a breast self-exam monthly. As women approach menopause, it's also a good idea to get a bone mineral density test. Men should receive an annual digital rectal exam if there is a strong family history of prostate cancer or if they are African-American, and a prostate specific antigen (PSA) test every year if they are at high risk. Men should also perform a testicular self-exam every month.

Fifties and Older

You should receive an eye exam every two to four years (and annually after age sixty-five), a fasting plasma glucose test every three years, a thyroid-stimulating hormone test every three to five years if sixty or older, a cholesterol test every five years (and every three years after age sixty), a fecal occult blood test annually, a sigmoidoscopy at age fifty, and a colonoscopy every ten years after that. You should also have your blood pressure checked at least once a year and preferably more often. Immunizations should include a pneumonia shot once after age sixty-five and a flu shot annually after age sixty-five or if you are in a high-risk group. Women should receive a pelvic exam annually, a Pap test every one to two years, and a clinical breast exam and mammogram annually, and they should perform a breast self-examination every month. Men should receive a digital rectal exam and a PSA test annually and perform a testicular self-exam monthly.

Customizing Your Personal Anti-aging Plan

Now that you've established that you're going to take a proactive approach toward anti-aging and you've found the physician that's right for you, it's time to plan, plan, plan. No single anti-aging regimen works for everyone. We all have different needs and goals, and these, rather than the "here today, gone tomorrow/everyone is doing it" fads, should determine your individual program.

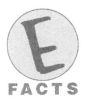

It's said that Cleopatra bathed in sour milk as part of her regular beauty regimen. This makes sense, since sour milk contains lactic acid—a weak chemical peel. Today, women buy a wide array of beauty creams that offer the same effect, but at considerably greater expense.

In an effort to help start you out, take a look at the following general outline designed to help you customize your personal anti-aging plan:

- *Identify your goals.* What do you hope to gain through your anti-aging regimen? Obviously, your primary goal will be to add as many active years to your life as possible. But what else do you hope to accomplish? A comprehensive but realistic list will go a long way toward helping you achieve your goals.
- *Develop a game plan.* Improving your health and adding years to your life isn't something that can be accomplished haphazardly. You need a workable plan—one you can live with. Reworking your entire life and making drastic lifestyle changes may look good on paper, but such a plan probably won't last long. Be realistic in what you hope to accomplish and how.

- *Do your homework.* Stay informed about what's currently available in anti-aging medicine and technology, as well as what the immediate future will hold. Pay particular attention to breakthroughs in nutrition, because that's where many researchers believe the key to longevity will be found. Talk with your physician about what you've read and learned and solicit his or her advice on what else you can do to improve and maintain your health.

- *Develop a healthy sense of skepticism.* As the baby boomers age, the demand for anti-aging innovations continues to grow stronger. A lot of products, particularly in the areas of cosmeceuticals and dietary supplements, are touted for their anti-aging effects, but there is no magic bullet. Anything that seems too good to be true almost certainly is. Spend your money only on what you know to be effective.

- *Eliminate bad habits.* If you smoke, quit. If you drink too much, stop or at least drink more moderately. If you aren't getting enough exercise, join a gym. If the only fruit and veggies in your kitchen are made of wax, make a concerted effort to add more fresh items to your daily diet. If you can't remember the last time you saw a doctor, make an appointment for a checkup. In short, do what you must to make your lifestyle more healthful in every way.

- *Know your genetic history.* Awareness of the chronic conditions or serious medical problems that have occurred in your family can often help you prevent them or, at the very least, prepare for their possibility. If you're unsure how older family members died, ask those who knew them or check their death certificates. At the very least, you should have this information on members of your immediate family—your parents, grandparents, siblings, aunts, uncles, first cousins, and so forth. But the farther back you can go in your ancestry, the better.

- *Enlist the aid of family and friends.* Slowing the aging process isn't something you have to do by yourself. Tell your family and friends of your plan and enlist their help in making it a reality. For example, if you're trying to kick the cigarette habit, ask them to not smoke in your presence. Or if you're trying to improve your nutrition, encourage them to try something more healthful than greasy fast food when dining out. You might also ask them to join you while you exercise. The physical activity will benefit everyone, and your chances of actually sticking with your exercise regimen increase when you participate with a partner. Most importantly, don't let anyone deride or ridicule your anti-aging regimen. There's nothing funny or pointless (no matter what your age) about trying to improve your health or add years to your life.

Aging Myths

Old age is a mystery to all but those who experience it. And as with all things unknown, there are several myths regarding old age. As you continue to perfect your anti-aging regimen, it's important to not let yourself get discouraged by false facts, figures, and stories. In fact, let's take a quick look at some of the most common aging myths and show you why they're incorrect.

Old Age Automatically Means Illness and Frailty

This may have been true in the past, but it's considerably less so today. A great many age-related diseases can now be treated to the point where quality of life is no longer affected. Thanks to advances in medical science and greater public education, the past three decades have seen a remarkable reduction in the prevalence of three important precursors to chronic illness: high blood pressure, high cholesterol, and smoking.

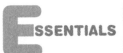

ESSENTIALS

One of the most common forms of discrimination in the United States is ageism. Like all forms of prejudice, ageism is based on false perceptions and gross generalizations. For example, while it's true that some older people drive poorly, most do not. Nor are all older people senile, sick, infirm, or stupid.

Old People Can't Learn Anything New

The rising number of seniors who are taking continuing education college courses just for the fun of it proves how untrue this adage really is. Nonetheless, many people still believe it, setting a trap for mental boredom and decay. The simple truth is that the majority of older people respond well to mental stimulation and enjoy learning new things.

Cosmeceuticals Work Like a Charm

As members of the baby boomer generation enter their forties and fifties, an increasing number are turning to pricey "cosmeceuticals"—cosmetics specially designed to prevent or eliminate wrinkles and other age-related skin blemishes—in an effort to maintain their youth.

Do these products work? Yes and no. They all contain essentially the same ingredients (antioxidants, copper peptides, moisturizers, hydroxy acids) but in varying amounts and combined with a wide variety of other ingredients. Many have been shown to eliminate fine lines on the face, but the effect is temporary and usually very subtle. Bottom line: Nothing that comes in a jar, no matter how much it costs, will get rid of deep wrinkles. For that, you need to consult a plastic surgeon.

Old Age Automatically Means a Descent into Senility

The stereotypical "demented geezer" is just that—a stereotype, and an incorrect stereotype at that. While many people do develop some form of senility in their later years, far more live out their lives with their mental faculties strong and intact. Mental acuity in our senior years is strongly dependent on regular stimulation, so it's important that you give your mind a mental workout every day.

Age-Related Health Problems Can't Be Reversed

Here's another false adage. Many of the health problems associated with old age can, in fact, be corrected with some simple lifestyle changes. Even lung damage from a lifetime of smoking can sometimes be improved just by kicking the habit. It's NEVER too late to reap the benefits of a healthy life!

Longevity Is Irreversibly Linked to Heredity

While it's true that a family history of longevity improves one's odds of living a long time, lifestyle, environment, and many other factors also play important roles. That's why people whose parents and grandparents died at a relatively young age shouldn't assume that they will die young as well. If these individuals take good care of themselves and pursue just some of the many anti-aging breakthroughs currently available, chances are very good that they'll be able to beat the odds.

Advancing Age Means an End to an Active Sex Life

The sexless senior citizen is an antiquated myth long dispelled by scientific and anecdotal research. Many seniors choose to give up an active sex life upon the passing of their mate, but the vast majority are able—and willing—to enjoy the many virtues of loving sex well into their seventies, eighties, and even older. As long as you remain physically healthy and mentally able, there's no reason to put sex on hold as you age.

CHAPTER 2

The Lowdown on Aging

Why do we age? Why does time take such a toll on the human body and mind? Why don't we mature to a certain age, then stop? These questions have perplexed researchers for centuries and continue to do so today. Scientists have a fairly good understanding of the physiology of aging—how time affects the body and mind on a cellular level—but there is still much debate within medical circles as to WHY we age. This chapter will take a look at the lowdown on aging.

The Human Machine

Though you may not think of it as such, the human body functions very much like a machine. The heart is its motor, and the food we eat is the fuel that drives it. As anyone who took high school physiology knows, our bodies are made up of billions of individual cells that comprise the various organs and systems, each with a unique but important function. Think of them as smaller machines working tirelessly within the whole.

Unlike most man-made machines, however, the human body never stops working; it operates every second of every minute of every hour for decade upon decade. In fact, it pumps blood through veins and capillaries, digests food, regulates hormones—the list of life-sustaining functions is endless—even while we sleep. And like any machine that works nonstop for sixty to seventy or more years, the human body eventually wears out. Cell reproduction slows or is altered, the exterior starts to show wear and tear, internal systems slowly begin to fail.

Such is aging.

This slow process affects everyone differently. Some people begin to show obvious signs of aging—thinning or graying hair, wrinkles on the face, leathery skin from too much sun exposure—at a relatively early age, sometimes even in their late teens and early twenties. Others age much more gracefully, appearing years, even decades, younger than they really are for their entire lives.

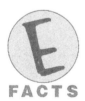

FACTS

According to a study conducted by the National Institute on Aging, there are approximately 35 million people in the United States age sixty-five or older, accounting for about 13 percent of the total population.

How and when aging affects us is a crapshoot that incorporates a wide range of factors, including genetics, environment, and lifestyle. The only universal truth is that we all will age.

However, like any machine, the lifespan of the human body can very often be extended through proper maintenance. Just as you must change your car's oil and give it a tune-up once in a while, so must the body be cared for and "tuned up" through proper nutrition, exercise, regular visits to the doctor, and other techniques. Simple common sense suggests that a body that is ignored over the course of its life is a body that will experience the ravages of age much more quickly than a body that is well cared for.

Theories of Aging

Wear and Tear Theory

One of the oldest theories of aging is the Wear and Tear Theory, first suggested in 1882 by a German biologist named Dr. August Weismann. Weismann believed that we showed signs of aging because of the use and abuse the body experiences over a lifetime. Some of this abuse is environmental (e.g., sun exposure, environmental toxins), and some of it is lifestyle (e.g., cigarette smoking, poor diet, alcohol consumption). Both combine to adversely affect the body's cells and organs over time until they simply can't function any more. When we're young, the body is able to repair damage to itself relatively easily. But as we age, this restorative ability becomes increasingly less effective.

The Neuroendocrine Theory

This concept carries the Wear and Tear Theory a step farther, concentrating on the neuroendocrine system—a complex network of essential biochemicals that stimulate the release of hormones and other compounds necessary to maintain life. Developed by Vladimir Dilman, Ph.D., this theory postulates that age causes the neuroendocrine system to gradually slow down, producing lower levels of the many hormones necessary for proper life function, as well as affecting the important interactions between them. The result is the physical effects commonly associated with aging, such as menopause, reduced muscle mass, and an increase in the risk and degree of degenerative disease. Based on this theory, many anti-aging programs include hormone replacement therapy as a way of reversing or postponing the effects of aging.

Age affects our metabolism in a number of ways. One of the most problematic is a reduced ability to absorb and metabolize drugs, which can adversely affect their efficacy. Worse, the majority of older people take more than one medication, increasing the risk of side effects or dangerous interactions.

The Genetic Control Theory

This theory suggests that we're the victims of planned obsolescence—that we're preprogrammed by our DNA to live only so long and then die. In short, our biological clock begins ticking from the moment we're born (actually, from the moment of conception), making old age and death an inescapable inevitability. However, everyone's genetic clock is set differently, so people age at different rates and show the signs of age in different ways. Lifestyle and environment are also believed to play a role in determining when our biological clocks go off.

Researchers who adhere to the Genetic Control Theory believe that the aging process can be slowed by using nutrition, drugs, and other compounds to protect and repair the DNA within our cells. In addition, gene therapy and/or gene manipulation may one day enable us to either stop the aging clock or repeatedly reset it—adding many years of healthy life.

The Free-Radical Theory

This currently is one of the most commonly accepted theories on why people age. It dates back to a concept first introduced in 1954 by a researcher named R. Gerschman and later developed by Dr. Denham Harman at the University of Nebraska College of Medicine. Much ongoing anti-aging research centers around the Free-Radical Theory and ways to keep free radicals from causing us harm.

Free radicals are unbalanced oxygen molecules containing an extra electron. Because nature likes equilibrium, free radicals are constantly searching for molecules to which they can attach and steal a matching electron. However, the theft of a matching electron only serves to create new free radicals in an ongoing process that ultimately results in cellular damage.

It's important to note, however, that free radical activity—a form of biochemical electricity—is not in itself bad. Without it, a great many important bodily functions, including hormone synthesis, smooth-muscle tone, and the maintenance of a strong immune system, would cease. Problems occur when free radicals attack cell membranes, inhibiting the cells' ability to reproduce or protect themselves. The effects of too many free radicals are many and include some of the better known signs of aging, including wrinkles, age spots, and poor skin quality. An abundance of free radicals can also lead to more serious problems, including cataracts, heart disease, and even the formation of certain kinds of cancer. Anti-aging researchers say that the answer can be found in chemicals known as antioxidants, which eat up excess free radicals.

The Waste Accumulation Theory

This concept is based on the fact that the body's cells produce more waste than they can get rid of over the course of their lifetime. This waste matter contains a variety of compounds, including poisons, which adversely affect cell function and eventually result in cell death when they reach a certain level. Over time, the effects of this ongoing cell destruction can be seen in the most common symptoms of aging.

The Cell Division Limitation Theory

This theory goes hand in hand with the Waste Accumulation Theory by speculating that the number of cell divisions is directly influenced by the buildup of cell waste. In short, the older we are, the more waste we accumulate. And the more waste we accumulate, the faster cells fall apart and the fewer times they can divide.

The Hayflick Limit Theory

Nearly forty years ago, two cell biologists, Hayflick and Moorehead, concluded that many types of cells are controlled by a special biological clock that limits their life span. For example, studies determined that human fibroblast cells, which are found in the lung, heart, muscle, and skin, divide approximately fifty times over the years and then stop. It was also noted that certain degenerations and other factors caused some cells to stop dividing before they were supposed to, theoretically resulting in the best-known indicators of age.

The Thymic-Stimulating Theory

The thymus gland, which is located in the base of the neck above the heart, plays an important role in the development of the immune system. Very large at birth, it gradually shrinks as we age, until it ceases to function. Some researchers theorize that the slow death of the thymus gland may be instrumental to the aging process by gradually weakening the immune system, and that "boosters" of thymic hormones may help slow the process by stimulating the production of certain neurotrans-mitters and hormones.

The Errors/Repairs Theory

This concept, developed in 1963 by researchers at the Salk Institute, hypothesizes that the physical signs of aging are the result of errors in the production of proteins and the reproduction of DNA within our cells. The body is usually able to make repairs naturally when problems arise in the reproduction of DNA, but it simply can't make perfect repairs every time. The result is an accumulation of imperfect molecules that can cause disease and other symptoms of aging.

The Autoimmune Theory

The immune system is our first and most effective line of defense against infection and disease. However, it becomes less efficient as we age, producing fewer disease-fighting antibodies. It also has a tendency to turn against itself, in essence attacking its own body. Common autoimmune diseases include rheumatoid arthritis, lupus, scleroderma, and adult-onset diabetes. It is also theorized that aging is an autoimmune response.

The Calorie Restriction Theory

This idea, first proposed by noted gerontologist Dr. Roy Walford of the UCLA Medical School, suggests that the effects of aging may actually be the result of too many calories over our lifetime. Through his studies, Walford concluded that a high-nutrient, low-calorie diet can have a dramatic effect in retarding the aging process by reducing weight to the point of metabolic efficiency. The downside is that the diet is very restricted.

The Telomerase Theory

This is the newest and one of the most promising theories regarding aging and possible ways to slow it down. Telomeres are sequences of nucleic acids that extend from the tips of our chromosomes. They help maintain chromosomal integrity and become a little bit shorter every time a cell divides. After a while, they become so short that the inevitable occurs: DNA damage and cellular death commonly associated with aging.

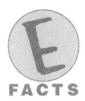

FACTS

Cancer cells thrive in the presence of the enzyme telomerase, which sustains the abnormal cell division that characterizes the disease. Tumor cells can be killed by turning off telomerase production, a treatment that has proved effective in several laboratory studies. Excited by these findings, researchers are now working on a drug or genetic therapy that effectively blocks telomerase and prevents cancer cells from dividing.

Researchers recently found that shrinking telomeres can be rebuilt with the help of the enzyme telomerase, which is found only in cancer cells and germ cells such as sperm. When telomerase was reactivated in laboratory tests, some normal cells experienced an almost indefinite life extension. Researchers are now trying to determine the exact influence of telomeres on the total aging process, and possible ways to synthesize the enzyme telomerase and use it to slow or prevent cellular damage and death.

The Physiology of Aging

The aging process is not something that suddenly kicks in on a given chronological date. It begins the moment we're born and continues, unrelenting, until we die. Its effects really start to become evident sometime between our twentieth and thirtieth birthdays and are increasingly obvious every year thereafter.

But what happens to us physiologically as we age? How does the process affect us cellularly, systematically, and as a complete organism? Researchers have studied this question for years and have a pretty good understanding of the general effects of age. Much of it is common knowledge, but some of it may surprise you.

Around age thirty, various systems begin a gradual decline. The immune system, for example, slowly becomes less and less efficient (putting us at greater risk of disease), and the muscular system begins to lose its tone (especially if we don't exercise regularly). The ratio of muscle to fat starts to decline around age thirty (and continues well into our eighties), with deposits of fat peaking around age fifty. Most of this fat accumulation occurs around the stomach, buttocks, and thighs. In addition, the abdomen begins to sag more because of the loss of muscle tone. Even our grip strength is affected, going from a high of 100 pounds at age thirty to around 75 pounds in our fifties and sixties.

Our metabolism begins to change (we gain weight easier and find it more difficult to lose), and our digestive tract, which used to be able to handle anything we popped into it, becomes sluggish and decidedly more sensitive. All of a sudden, our favorite dinner of tacos and chilies washed down with a pitcher of beer is no longer the fast fuel it used to be. At the same time, a decrease in glucose tolerance increases the risk of developing diabetes (especially if we're overweight), and increased blood pressure puts us at greater risk of heart disease (especially if we add a lot of salt to our food).

Indeed, the heart experiences some important changes as we age. Once we pass our fortieth birthday, the heart muscle may enlarge so it can pump more blood as it tries to compensate for clogged and hardening arteries. At the same time, the covering sheath around the heart may thicken, resulting in an overall reduction in blood output. This decrease leads to a decline in the supply of oxygen to muscle tissue, in turn resulting in a reduction in aerobic capacity. Bottom line: Even minimal exercise hits us harder and tires us more quickly.

Our lungs feel the effects of aging, too, gradually losing their elasticity until, by age fifty, breath capacity is 20 percent less than what it was when we were twenty. Of course, smokers lose breath capacity much faster than nonsmokers, in addition to placing themselves as greater risk of emphysema, lung cancer, and other pulmonary ailments.

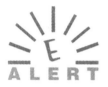

Roller coasters are a fun fright, but they can be hazardous to your health. According to researchers, repeated roller-coaster rides can result in dangerous blood clots on the surface of the brain—a condition that can lead to brain damage, seizures, and even death.

Skin tone and elasticity begins to break down in our twenties as collagen decreases, though the rate at which our skin ages is determined by a number of factors, including family history, lifestyle, and environment. People who spent a great deal of their youth in the sun develop weathered skin (and a greater risk of skin cancer) more quickly than those who took precautions. Thinning of the outer layers causes the skin to begin sagging around age fifty, and both sun damage and clumping pigment cells, known as melanocyte cells, result in so-called liver spots and other unsightly blotches. The skin also becomes dryer, resulting in a greater need for moisturizers, as well as more prone to bruising.

The effects of aging are also seen in the hair. Oil glands in the scalp begin to dry out as we grow older, causing our hair to become brittle and more easily broken. And one of the most common indicators of age—white or graying hair—occurs when the hair cells gradually stop producing pigment. Researchers have found that nearly half of men and women of European descent will have at least some noticeable graying by age fifty, if not a complete head of gray hair, and those of non-European extraction can expect to see some "silver threads among the gold" about a decade later, if not before. When it comes to hair, men have it worse than women; nearly half of all men can expect some balding by their fiftieth birthday.

The brain is also affected by age. Researchers note that the brain tends to shrink an average of 6 percent over our lifetime, resulting in a loss of cognitive abilities such as memory, problem solving, and digesting information. Forgetfulness is, without question, one of the most common "complaints" of aging, though it's more often due to reduced oxygen or a lack of use than to Alzheimer's disease or other organic disorders. Indeed, the phrase "use it or lose it" really applies to the brain; studies have found that older individuals who enjoy solving puzzles, read a lot, or regularly engage in other forms of mental stimulation tend to have better memories than those who don't.

The advancing years take their toll on the senses as well, especially smell and taste, which are very closely linked to our enjoyment of food. Taste buds in the mouth and olfactory receptors in the nose become increasingly less sensitive, which is why many older people complain that eating is no longer the pleasurable experience it once was. (This also explains why a lot of older people eat less than they did when they were younger.) Like most other indicators of age, a diminishing sense of taste and smell may also be affected by a nutritional deficiency, such as of zinc, and environment and lifestyle factors—especially smoking.

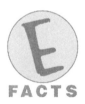

FACTS

Vision is one of the most advanced sensory systems in the human body. Our eyes are uniquely designed to receive visual images, but it's the brain that interprets and processes these images and determines whether we should react to them, ignore them, or store them in memory for later recall.

Vision, too, fares poorly as we age. A loss of elasticity in the eye's lens often results in presbyopia (an age-related inability to focus on objects that are near), and night blindness may become more pronounced due to a slow loss of photoreceptors in the retina. In addition, older people often find it difficult to differentiate between colors, particularly in the yellow-blue color spectrum, because the cornea (the clear lens over the pupil) thickens and becomes somewhat yellowish in color. Age also makes us more prone to a variety of other vision disorders, including cataracts, glaucoma, diabetic retinopathy, and macular degeneration. Dry-eye is a common complaint among many older people because of diminishing tear production, and there may also be a wrinkling and loosening of the skin around the eyelids due to loss of tone and decreased elasticity of the eyelid muscle. In addition, a loss of orbital fat often causes the eyes to sink deeper into the skull, limiting upward gaze.

Hearing tends to peak at puberty, and gradually declines after that, though many baby boomers no doubt hastened their hearing loss with too much loud music when they were younger. In fact, hearing experts anticipate a dramatic increase in hearing problems among boomers fifty and younger, due to a lack of precautions during their teens, twenties, and thirties. Generally speaking, a sensitivity to the higher tones is the first to go, particularly among men. Nutrition, environment, occupation, and other factors can also play a role in hearing loss as we age.

A measurable loss in bone density and mineral content is also a common sign of aging. Brittle bones due to low calcium levels—a condition known as osteoporosis—tend to afflict women more commonly than men, especially after menopause, though men are certainly at risk. In addition to breaking more easily, older bones have greater difficulty mending. The regular consumption of calcium over one's lifetime is the best and easiest way to maintain bone strength during our later years, but most people don't even think about it until it's too late.

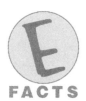

FACTS

Our senses become increasingly less sensitive as we age. Studies suggest that up to 40 percent of people eighty years and older have difficulty identifying common substances by smell.

Even our urinary tracts are affected by age. Around age thirty, the kidneys begin to shrink in size and function less efficiently, and the bladder begins to lose its elasticity, requiring more frequent urination. Urinary incontinence is a common complaint among the elderly, afflicting an estimated 20 percent of older people living at home and 75 percent living in long-term care facilities. Sometimes urinary incontinence can be corrected through surgery, Kegel exercises, or biofeedback, though many older people are reluctant to seek help for this embarrassing and socially isolating problem.

Finally, there's sex. In the eyes of many—including too many physicians—the elderly are a sexless population that no longer desire or pursue regular intimacy. However, numerous studies have found this to be completely untrue; the majority of older people continue to enjoy a healthy and fulfilling sex life well into their seventies, eighties, and beyond.

Still, the passing years do result in some changes. Most women experience menopause around age fifty, when their estrogen level plummets and ovulation comes to an end. The lack of estrogen in the system often results in thinning of the vaginal tissue and reduced lubrication during arousal, all of which can make intercourse painful if precautions, such as the use of a commercial lubricant, are not taken. Some women also experience a loss of libido following menopause, though others say their sex drives have never been stronger. Obviously, it depends on the individual.

Men experience numerous age-related changes in sexual function as well. After age forty, the strength of their erections gradually begins to decrease, as does the volume and intensity of their ejaculations. Older men also require more time to "rest up" between sexual encounters and may experience a loss of libido and other problems due to a deficiency of testosterone or other hormones (men's testosterone levels drop by nearly 40 percent in the five decades between ages thirty and eighty). In both sexes, pubic hair may turn gray or start to thin with age, though this has no effect on sexual functioning.

The Psychological Effects of Aging

Entire books have been written on the psychology of aging, an aspect that most researchers now consider just as important as physiology when discussing the process and ways to slow it down. The reason: How you mentally approach the passage of time has a lot to do with how happy and active you will be in your later years.

Of course, a tremendous number of factors come into play in determining our psychological attitude as we age. Take health, for example. People who are in good health and free of age-related diseases will almost certainly enjoy their later years far more than those who are chronically ill. The latter individuals may find themselves spending their twilight years in chronic pain, financially burdened, and with dwindling social support. Sadly, a great many of this nation's long-term care facilities are full of such people, once young and vital, now bedridden, simply waiting for the clock to run out.

Financial status can also play an important role in our psychological view of aging. Older people with an adequate expendable income have much more freedom than those who are on a fixed income, and this situation can have a dramatic impact on whether individuals view their senior years as a time of travel, adventure, and knowledge or as a time of poverty, reduced activity, and dwindling social interaction. Obviously, those in the latter category would be less inclined and less able to pursue anti-aging technologies or lifestyle changes than those in the former category.

Equally important to the psychological component of aging is social support. In years past, families were typically larger and more extended. Older family members lived with loved ones and contributed to the family good by caring for children and sharing the wisdom that comes with age. Older people also tended to have a stronger friendship base, socializing frequently with neighbors and acquaintances they had known for decades.

But the concept of the close-knit extended family changed dramatically in the 1950s and 1960s, when Americans began spreading their wings in increasing numbers, packing up everything they had and moving to new and more prosperous locales. Older members were often "dumped" in rest homes or left to fend for themselves in the old neighborhood.

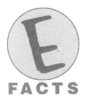

FACTS

Memories tend to be less clear than perceptions, though occasionally a memory will be so vivid as to include virtually every detail. This phenomenon is known as eidetic imagery, and is most commonly found in children.

The sad result of this national exodus is that social interaction and support—an extremely vital component of successful and happy aging—has, in many cases, become increasingly difficult to find and maintain. Many seniors, especially those who are widowed, spend their days alone, afraid, and depressed. It's no way to live the final years of one's life, yet tens of thousands of Americans do it, despite the best efforts of churches and social agencies. As might be expected, older individuals who spend their days doing nothing more than watching television and waiting desperately for the phone to ring are not eager to face tomorrow, much less the next five or ten or twenty years. Existing but not living, many depressed seniors choose to take their own lives.

Of course, it's easy—and incorrect—to paint too gloomy a picture of aging. The truth is that much of what we believe about old age is now outdated, stereotypical, or just plain wrong. For example, advancing age does not have to mean illness and infirmity; breakthroughs in medical science now allow us to live longer and better than ever before. Indeed, many medical conditions that in the past meant years of chronic pain or immobility can now be completely eliminated or at least treated to the point where they no longer impact quality of life. In addition, proper financial planning during middle age can guarantee sufficient income after retirement, and numerous support organizations, clubs, and agencies for seniors can help make sure that no one spends their days lonely and depressed.

A recent report from the National Institute on Aging, titled *Older Americans 2000: Key Indicators of Well-Being,* revealed some startling changes in the quality of life experienced by most older Americans. Among its findings:

- Life expectancy for Americans age sixty-five in 2000 is another eighteen years, on average. In 1900, sixty-five-year-olds could expect to live only another twelve years.
- From 1959 to 1998, the percentage of older Americans living in poverty declined from 35 percent to 11 percent.
- The median net worth in households headed by older people increased from 1984 to 1999 by 70 percent, but there is a startling disparity between races. In 1999, the median net worth in households headed by older blacks was $13,000, compared to $181,000 for older whites.

- Heart disease, cancer, and stroke are the three big killers. Mortality rates for heart disease and stroke have declined by a third since 1980, while the rate for cancer has gone up slightly.
- The rate of chronic disability among older Americans declined from 24 percent in 1982 to 21 percent in 1994.
- A survey of Americans age sixty-five and older between 1994 and 1996 found that the majority considered themselves healthy.

For a growing number of people, the senior years are seen as a time of excitement, because they mean freedom and opportunity. Child rearing is over, they're comfortably retired, and they have everything to look forward to. In short, they're psychologically comfortable with a process they can't stop but can, in many ways, help control. It's these people who look at anti-aging research with hope, eager to add more years to their life as well as more life to their years.

The Effects of Personality on Aging

The effect personality has on the aging process cannot be overstated. Our personality determines our emotional and psychological state, which in turn has a very strong influence on our health. And when our health turns sour, we can practically feel the years being taken away from us.

Type-A personalities are most at risk, say behavior experts. They tend to be aggressive, forceful, take-charge individuals who want immediate results, and they aren't afraid to push themselves and their employees like lapdogs in order to get them. Anger and rage are not uncommon emotions among type-A personalities, which no doubt explains why so many of them keel over from a heart attack at an unusually early age. These men and women make very effective corporate executives, but the constant stress and pressure on which they thrive can take a heavy toll, especially if you add a lifetime of poor diet, lack of exercise, and other similar factors.

If you have a type-A personality, don't expect to live to a ripe old age. Stress and negative emotions can have a potentially deadly impact on every aspect of your health, weakening your immune system and placing you at increased risk of a wide variety of ailments.

The answer? Slow down and smell the roses. Reduce your workload, delegate authority, and take some time off. Start meditating, get more exercise, and do whatever else you must to reduce the stress in your life. The results will amaze you. You'll be happier and healthier, and you'll slow down the aging process.

The Emotional Effects of Aging

The phenomenon of aging evokes a wide range of emotions throughout our entire lives. In our youth, we view the process of growing older with excitement, anticipation, and wonder. When we're nine years old, it seemingly takes forever to reach 10. So anxious are we to advance another year that we start counting in increments—9¼, 9½, 9¾. The anticipation grows even stronger when we're in our teens, especially if there's the promise of a new car on our next birthday. But, in a humorous analogy to Einstein's Theory of Relativity, when we're forty-nine, that dreaded fiftieth birthday seems to be upon us in the blink of an eye, no matter how hard we try to ignore it.

Old age shouldn't have too much of an impact on people in good physical and mental health. As long as older individuals are also financially secure and have a strong social support base, they can expect to remain relatively happy, content, and joyful no matter how many years they have under their belts.

Unexpected and unwanted physical and cognitive changes, however, can result in a wide array of negative emotions, including fear, anxiety, depression, anger, and even rage. This is especially true among people who find themselves afflicted with chronic illness, impaired mobility, and/or dwindling social support. All of this is understandable, say psychologists; no one wants to watch the beauty and vigor of youth slowly give way to an increasingly nonfunctioning body or mind, not to mention the loss of independence that often goes with it.

The physical effects of aging can be devastating, as well as financially and emotionally costly. But the loss of cognitive function from age-related dementia is often more so. Many forms of dementia are slow to develop, giving the afflicted person plenty of time to dwell on his or her bleak future. Not surprisingly, this often leads to incapacitating depression and a host of other negative emotions that, in turn, can have serious physical consequences as well. (There's no question that our emotions are directly linked to our physical well-being; anyone who doesn't believe that high stress can have physical manifestations simply has never experienced it.) During times such as these, loving support from family, friends, and clergy is vital to helping older people maintain their emotional strength and equilibrium.

Since human beings are not robots, the emotional component of aging must be an important part of all anti-aging research. The goal must be not only added years in good physical health but also strong psychological and emotional health as well. One cannot be achieved without the other two.

Until very recently, a noticeable decline in mental function was considered a normal part of aging. The older you were, the more "senile" you were expected to become. Even doctors felt this way, often dismissing elderly patients concerned about their diminished mental skills with the comment, "There's nothing we can do about it, so you might as well accept it." This offhand, often inaccurate diagnosis typically left patients angry and sad; after a vital, healthy life, they were suddenly doomed to an existence of mental decay for which there was no hope of recovery.

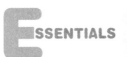
SSENTIALS

Maintaining mental acuity throughout your life requires some effort on your part. After all, nothing stays strong without sufficient exercise. Use brain games to help keep your memory and other cognitive functions in peak condition. For example, read a short passage from a book three times, then try to write the passage from memory.

Today, of course, we know that the stereotypical "demented old geezer" is more myth than medical fact. Old age doesn't automatically mean a substantial loss of memory or other cognitive skills any more than it automatically means heart disease, cancer, or any other supposedly age-related medical condition. Numerous studies have concluded that mental acuity can remain strong even at the 100-year mark and offer as proof the tens of thousands of Americans who have stayed bright and sharp witted well into their senior years.

The last few decades have shed tremendous light on how age affects the brain and how we can keep our mental faculties sharp regardless of the number of years under our belts. Senility is not a forgone conclusion for anyone; many common types of mental degeneration are the result of lifestyle more than age and very often can be reversed with a simple change in diet or medication. This is great news for people looking to add years to their lives, since dementia has long been considered a stubborn obstacle in the quest for greater longevity.

This isn't to suggest, of course, that dementia in its varied forms should not be an important concern for older adults. Awareness of the risk of dementia and its early indicators allows those afflicted to take advantage of early treatment, which often can slow its progress.

The loss of mental function has become a national issue, thanks to medical advances that now allow people with chronic disorders such as Alzheimer's disease to live far longer than they did in the past. As a result, the majority of Americans are now either caring for an affected loved one or know someone who is.

Indeed, our nursing homes and long-term care facilities are overwhelmed with people afflicted with Alzheimer's disease and other forms of mental degeneration. And these numbers are expected to increase dramatically in coming years as baby boomers enter their senior years.

Concurrently, our health care system must also deal with the growing number of Americans who suddenly find themselves having to care for loved ones who, while often physically healthy, can no longer care for themselves due to dementia. The financial burden of elder care can be devastating, as can the physical and mental toll experienced by family caregivers. Many are members of the so-called "sandwich generation," caring for both children and ailing parents or grandparents, so it's not surprising that so many eventually fall victim to stress-related health problems that impact on their own longevity.

In the following sections, we will continue to discuss how age affects the brain and what you can do to maintain your mental acuity through your middle and senior years.

Your Brain: Use It or Lose It

The brain isn't a muscle, but it still needs to be exercised in order to achieve peak performance. Failure to stimulate cognitive function on a regular basis can actually lead to mental impairment. In other words, use it or lose it.

FACTS

Surely you've heard the idea that we use just 10 percent of our brains. The exact number of neurons in the human brain is unknown. Because of this, it is impossible to determine exactly how many cells are involved in any particular function and, thus, impossible to determine what percentage of the brain is being used at any given time.

Numerous studies have shown that people who lead lives with little mental stimulation experience greater cognitive loss as they age. Their memory fails with greater frequency, and they find it increasingly difficult to work puzzles, perform mathematic equations, and do other mental feats that come quite easily to people who "exercise" their brains often.

The reasons behind a lack of mental stimulation are many. Some people become numbed by too much television, while others dull their brains with alcohol and other stupefying substances. Prescription and over-the-counter drug interactions can also impair cognitive function, as can certain medical conditions. But for the majority of older Americans, isolation and a lack of social interaction are the primary culprits.

This makes perfect sense when you think about it. Social support means a lot of social interaction. We chat with friends, engage in a variety of activities, and live a relatively active life. All of this stimulates the brain on a number of important levels, keeping our cognitive skills well honed. But older people who lack social support often have little to do to occupy their time except watch television. Opportunities to actually think, to exercise the brain, become increasingly limited. And with this lack of stimulation comes a subtle but serious reduction in mental functioning.

Older people who find themselves less than mentally stimulated needn't despair. Clinical studies have demonstrated that brain function can be dramatically improved when exposed to greater cognitive stimulation regardless of a person's age. All you have to do is take the initiative. Turn off the television and read a book. Take up a challenging hobby. Engage friends in a lively debate on the issues of the day. Go to museums. Attend lectures. Work the crossword puzzle in the daily newspaper.

In other words, give your brain a workout every day. The harder you push it, the better it will perform.

The Brain: A User's Manual

If you're going to keep your brain functioning well throughout your life, it's important that you know how it works. Most people take their brains for granted, never fully comprehending the enormity of this astounding organ's ability and function.

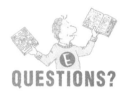

QUESTIONS?

Why does your heart beat and your lungs take in air without your having to tell them to?
Your autonomic nervous center takes care of it for you. Heart function and breathing are just two of the many reflexive activities governed by the autonomic nervous center. Others include the digestive system, the operation of certain glands, and maintenance of the body's internal environment.

Virtually every aspect of your existence—physical, mental, and emotional—is governed by the 3-pound mass of pinkish gray tissue safely encased within your skull. It enables you to live and survive, and it makes you who you are in every sense. If your heart or liver fails, you can get another one. If you lose an arm or a leg, you can get a prosthesis. But if anything happens to your brain, you'll most likely be left either incapacitated or dead. That's why it's so important that you take good care of your brain, protect it at all costs, and keep it stimulated for optimum performance. Once it's gone, so are you.

Fascinating Brain Tricks

One of the most noticeable things about the human brain is its symmetry. The two hemispheres fit nicely together, and one would assume that the organ's function is symmetrical as well. However, researchers have found that this isn't the case. Each hemisphere performs unique and specialized functions and dominates the other when it comes to specific jobs. This dominance, studies have found, is directly related to whether a person is right-handed or left-handed. In most right-handed people, the left hemisphere processes language, speech, and math skills, while the right hemisphere interprets complex imagery and spatial relationships and recognizes and regulates emotion. In left-handed people, brain organization is somewhat more variable.

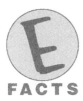

FACTS

Within the animal kingdom, evolution plays a big role in determining which parts of the brain are more developed. Birds, for example, often require amazing visual acuity to spot food on the ground while they are flying high above, so their optic lobes and cerebellum are often extremely well developed. Small nocturnal rodents, however, tend to have somewhat less developed frontal lobes because they rely more on other sensory systems such as smell and hearing for survival.

Hemispheric specialization has been difficult to study. Most breakthroughs have come from research on individuals who have experienced damage to the connections between the two hemispheres as a result of stroke or other medical conditions that destroy the nerve cells in that region. Much information has also been obtained from patients who have had to have the hemispheres surgically separated to control epilepsy, a serious neurological condition that can cause seizures.

Over the years, scientists have relied on two approaches to help them understand how the brain works. The first approach looks at brain function after a part of the brain has been damaged by disease or injury.

Functions that no longer work or that work differently after a brain injury shed tremendous light on how the brain operates and on what parts of the brain are responsible for specific functions or behaviors.

The second approach involves directly stimulating parts of the brain or analyzing brain function during sensory stimulation. Magnetic resonance imaging (MRI), electroencephalography (EEG), positron emission tomography (PET), and other technologies have been of tremendous assistance in brain research because they can document such things as blood flow, oxygen consumption, and glucose metabolism in the brain during specific functions or monitor electrical activity—the brain's unique "language"—when certain senses are activated. But despite these advances in technology, much of what the brain does (and how it does it) still defies explanation.

Age and Information

We live in an era of rapid information processing. Never before in human history has so much data been so readily available and at such a remarkable rate. This is good news for high school and college students, but less so for their parents and grandparents. The reason? Age takes a toll on our ability to assimilate or process information quickly. In short, it takes our brains a little longer to understand new information and put it to use. In addition, age appears to affect certain types of memory, which can also influence our information processing skills.

Researchers have yet to fully figure out what happens within the brain to reduce our information processing and memory skills. One theory suggests that the age-related loss of neurons affects cognitive processing by forcing information to take a somewhat circuitous route through the brain.

Can this have an adverse impact on quality of life? Well, it can—but only in extreme cases. The detectable but relatively mild impairment of information processing rarely affects the day-to-day life of the average senior simply because daily activities usually don't require us to assimilate and react to information immediately. We process it at our leisure and react to it as necessary. Besides, the mental processing of information is only one part of cognitive function, and certainly not the most important. So don't worry too much if it takes you a little longer to "get it." You may need to be a little more patient when engaging in your favorite mental pursuits, but you'll still get them done and with the same degree of enjoyment.

Maintaining Mental Acuity

Keeping the brain strong and nimble isn't a quest just for seniors; it's something we should strive for throughout our lives. By exercising our brain on a regular basis while we're young, we all but guarantee that cognitive function will remain in top form into our seventies, eighties, and beyond.

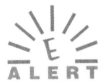

Every day, it seems, scientists uncover new and stronger evidence that vitamins and minerals play an integral role in slowing the aging process. Ask your doctor what you should be taking every day, and try to stay current with the most recent research.

Among older people, memory is the most commonly affected cognitive ability. Everyone's mind goes blank now and then. (How many times have you stood in the middle of a room, having completely forgotten why you are there?) But for many people, these so-called "senior moments" occur with frightening regularity. If this sounds like you, don't panic; your experiences are completely normal and easy to fix with a little effort.

According to researchers, older people are particularly prone to losing what's known as explicit memory—the ability to remember and later recall a particular name, date, or other fact on demand. This often occurs when trying to recall the name of a close friend or a vacation spot you've visited for years. The information is well known and on the tip of your tongue, but you just can't quite get it. Inevitably, this information will flash in your brain a few minutes later, after you've ceased struggling to grasp it.

What's interesting is that other types of memory usually don't decline with age. Working memory—the learned routines that get us through the day—remains particularly strong, as does long-term memory. In fact, long-term memory is usually the last to go, as often demonstrated by older individuals afflicted with dementia in the form of Alzheimer's disease.

The most striking area in which older people and younger people differ is in how they remember. In general, younger people are more adept at learning and retaining information in the face of distractions such as television, loud music, or crowds. Their brains, it seems, are better at multitasking, that is, engaging in several functions at once, such as watching a movie on TV while cramming for a history exam. Older people, as a rule, require a more quiet environment in which to digest new information for later retrieval.

Studies have concluded that this dramatic generational difference in learning and memorizing is due to the fact that older people have greater difficulty filtering out useless stimuli, such as music or conversation. Their brains absorb everything, affecting the memorization of pertinent information. For this reason, seniors are encouraged to read or study in a quiet environment, where they won't be easily distracted and can focus on the task at hand.

Other cognitive problems often experienced by older people include difficulty understanding or completing math problems, and difficulty figuring out visual-spatial puzzles. While sometimes a sign of early dementia, these problems most often are simply the result of mental inactivity, of not sufficiently exercising the brain in these particular areas.

Maintaining mental acuity is like training to be a professional athlete; you must pursue it full time and with all the energy you have. The future results are too important for this to be a half-hearted venture. The key is training and practice. You must treat your brain like a muscle, giving it a workout on a regular basis.

Research has proved the success of training and practice when it comes to maintaining and strengthening our mental abilities. In one study, scientists evaluated the number of words people could recall after listening to a lengthy list of random words. Before they received memory training, the older members of the study group were able to recall fewer words than the younger members. But after just a handful of memory training sessions, which included tips such as placing words in meaningful groups rather then trying to memorize them out of context, the older participants were able to triple their word recall.

What can you do to maintain cognitive function? Plenty. Here are some general tips:

- Enhance your memorization at every opportunity and take advantage of the challenges life presents every day. For example, when introduced to someone new, repeat the person's name to yourself three times and use it in conversation. See how well you remember the name the next morning.

- Another memory trick is to turn a grocery run into a game. After you've made a written list of your needs, memorize it to the best of your ability by taking a mental walk through your kitchen and pantry. Shop without referring to the list and see how well you've done before checking out. If your memory is sharp, you'll probably be able to remember almost everything.

- Stimulate your brain by doing puzzles, such as the daily crossword puzzle, anagrams, find-a-word, and maze games. Puzzles are a great way to strengthen and maintain several different areas of cognitive function, including memory and visual-spatial areas. Puzzle books can be purchased very inexpensively and are a great way to kill time while waiting in line or for an appointment.

- Read as much as you can and focus on works that challenge you. The latest potboiler may be a fun read, but it's probably as mentally challenging as a Dick and Jane primer. You can give your brain a workout by reading a literary classic you've always meant to tackle or by reading a nonfiction book on a topic you're interested in but know nothing about. Read carefully, with memory and recall in mind. To help you assimilate this new information, discuss it with friends.

- Take continuing education classes. Education is never a bad thing, and studies have shown that the more education you receive, the better your mental acuity—and the longer you will retain it. Take a class that challenges your thought processes, rather than something with which you're already familiar. Most community colleges and universities offer continuing education classes on a wide variety of subjects, and many sessions are held at night to accommodate people who work during the day.

- Teach a continuing education class. In addition to the joy that comes with sharing your life wisdom, teaching helps strengthen mental function through reading, self-learning, and lecturing. Everyone is adept at something, so choose your specialty, approach a local continuing education program, and improve the world with your knowledge. You don't need a teaching degree, just experience.

- Learn a foreign language. Being multilingual is extremely beneficial these days, and learning a foreign language can also be quite mentally challenging because it requires the thoughtful assimilation of new information and a strong memory. Once you've learned a new language, reward yourself with a vacation to another country so that you can practice.

- Start a hobby that requires coordination between multiple brain regions, such as dancing, painting, or learning a musical instrument. All of these strengthen and maintain mental acuity on a variety of levels.

- Improve your mathematic abilities by doing calculations in your head whenever possible. For example, balance your checkbook without the aid of a calculator and mentally figure out sales tax and how much change you should get back whenever you make a purchase. Reliance on technology tends to dull our math skills, a situation that only worsens with age.

- Write your autobiography. This can be a very rewarding activity in that you preserve your life experiences for the benefit of other family members and exercise your brain in the process. Recalling previous events requires a strong memory (which may be aided by going through photo albums, letters, etc.), and the act of writing improves visual-spatial skills. If you've lived a truly extraordinary life, consider getting your memoirs published.

CHAPTER 3

Exercise and Nutrition

How integral to your lifestyle are issues of health? Do you take nutrition into consideration when planning your weekly menu, or is convenience the most important factor? Do you make a concerted effort to exercise at least four times a week? While a growing number of Americans work hard at improving and maintaining their health, most of us really don't think that much about it until we get sick and need to see a doctor. And that's not good, especially from an anti-aging perspective.

Living a Healthful Lifestyle

Our lifestyle—the way we live our lives on a daily basis—plays a far greater role in determining how we'll age and how long we'll live than most of us understand. Every day, we make decisions big and small that impact on our health, right down to the cellular level. Some of these decisions, such as having fresh fruit for dessert instead of an entire chocolate cake, improve our health and thus our longevity. Others can cause or exacerbate health problems that may not be revealed for years or even decades.

The decision to live a healthful lifestyle is one only you can make. No one can force you to live more healthfully, to give up those habits that you know are bad for you and start others that promise to add years to your life. Doctors suggest, and family members nag; but in the end, it's your decision and yours alone.

Think about it. What changes could you make today that will improve your health tomorrow and for years to come? Take a moment right now to honestly evaluate your lifestyle and ask yourself that hard question. You'll probably be surprised at how many "bad" things you do on a regular basis and how many "good" things you could add. For example, analyze your exercise regimen—if you have one. Unfortunately, most of us cringe at the thought of our minimal exercise and our not-so-nutritional diets. Take a minute to think about that diet. Is it something your doctor would approve of?

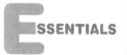

Doctors have long touted the effectiveness of an exercise/diet combo when it comes to losing weight, and a recent study confirms it. Bottom line: Exercising while you diet helps you stick to your diet regimen, according to the *American Journal of Clinical Nutrition*.

Exercise and nutrition are two of the most important variables when taking a proactive approach toward anti-aging. In this chapter, we're going to take a closer look at how you can make exercise work for you, as well as how your diet may add several years to your life.

Don't look at changing your lifestyle as a chore. Instead, look at it as an opportunity to do something tremendously beneficial for yourself and for your loved ones. Remember, it's never too late to make changes. Every bad habit you drop and every good habit you pick up can only improve your health and, in the long run, help you age with strength and vigor. Start slowly and involve your family. Change occurs more easily when you have a strong and loving support system.

The Importance of Exercise

Man was not created to live a sedentary lifestyle, yet that's what too many of us do. We need exercise to stay healthy, and we need it throughout our lives—not just when we're young or in middle age. In fact, seniors need regular physical activity just as much as younger people, if not more.

The benefits of exercise, regardless of age, are many. Regular physical activity keeps our muscles toned and strong, helps us maintain our ideal weight by burning calories, maintains bone strength and density, and improves and maintains heart and lung function. For example, simply taking a thirty-minute walk every day can reduce your risk of heart attack after just five months, doctors report. Exercise also builds stamina, improves flexibility, boosts our immune system, makes sex more fun, reduces our risk of cancer, improves our reflexes, lowers stress, and benefits our overall physical and mental health.

In addition, exercise helps keep our metabolism functioning at maximum capacity, which becomes increasingly important as we age. Why? Our metabolism slows with each passing year, making it increasingly difficult to process fatty acids. This, in turn, affects almost all of the body's systems, diminishing immune response and increasing our risk of atherosclerotic disease.

Exercise can be divided into three specific types: general activity, activities to build stamina, and exercises to increase strength and flexibility. All three are important to health and aging and should be integrated into your workout regimen.

General exercise includes any activity that requires the use of muscles, such as walking around the block, doing housework or yard work, and taking the stairs at work rather than the elevator. This is the most basic form of exercise and the easiest to do regardless of age. And while you may not break much of a sweat, the benefits are many. Among other things, general physical activity helps keep the muscles toned and helps maintain your ideal weight by burning extra calories.

Exercises that increase stamina greatly benefit the heart and lungs. These activities involve far more exertion than general physical activity and include such things as running, cycling, swimming, tennis, and racquetball. The goal is to strengthen the heart and lungs by working both at full capacity. If you haven't exercised in a while, it's a good idea to start slowly and gradually increase the amount of exercise you do in a week. As your stamina increases, you'll find it easier to do more and more. If you're over forty, it's also wise to get a physical exam from your doctor before starting any type of stamina-building exercise—just to be on the safe side.

Exercises to increase strength and flexibility include weight lifting (whether through the use of free weights or the kind of weight machines found in most gyms), yoga, and similar stretching activities. Maintaining strength, muscle tone, and flexibility is especially important during our middle and senior years, and there are additional benefits as well, such as improving bone density and reducing risk of injury from accidents. Weight-bearing exercises are particularly important for women because they can help prevent the onset of osteoporosis later in life by maintaining bone density before, during, and after menopause. And you don't have to lift weights until you bulge like Mr. Universe; most health specialists say thirty to forty minutes of weight training a week is sufficient to maintain optimum health.

If you want to age well and add many more active and vibrant years to your life, it's important that you incorporate all three aspects of exercise into your lifestyle. Begin by evaluating your daily routine to see where you can incorporate more physical activity. For example, you can do the following:

- Rather than sitting in the lunchroom, grab a low-cal sandwich and walk around the block during your lunch hour.
- Take a walk around the block every evening before dinner.
- Take the stairs instead of the elevator whenever possible.
- Park your car in the back of the lot and walk the extra distance to the store.
- If you play golf, walk the course rather than ride in a golf cart.

- Turn your housework routine into a workout routine by doing it to music.
- Play with your children in the backyard.
- Join a softball or other intramural sports team.
- Take the dog for a run rather than a walk.

Many people find that joining a gym gives them the incentive they need to perform aerobic and strength-building exercises, but it's not absolutely necessary. However, if you do decide to exercise at home, try do so with an exercise buddy. Studies have shown that people who exercise with someone else are less likely to give up early and more likely to enjoy the activities they perform. Effective stamina-building activities include the following:

- Running or jogging
- Cycling
- Swimming laps in a pool
- Playing tennis, racquetball, or handball
- Performing heart-pumping aerobic exercises to music
- Inline skating

Weight lifting can also be done at home. Inexpensive hand weights in various sizes can be purchased at any sporting goods store, but if you don't have any, gallon jugs filled with varying amounts of water make a good substitute. Start with a fairly low weight and gradually add on more as your strength increases. And don't push yourself too fast; overexertion with weights can cause serious injury.

One last reminder: Consult your doctor before engaging in any strenuous exercise regimen, especially if it's been a long time since you last exercised. A physical exam can detect heart and other health problems that could be made worse with intense physical activity.

Exercise and Longevity

The influence of exercise on longevity isn't just theory. Several clinical studies have shown a definitive link between regular exercise and longer life. In one of the most telling, Dr. Ralph Paffenbarger and colleagues monitored almost 17,000 Harvard male alumni with very similar demographic characteristics and found that those who expended fewer than 500 calories a week on exercise had the highest death rate. Those who used up between 500 and 1,000 calories a week on exercise (the equivalent of walking between 5 and 10 miles, respectively) had a 22 percent lower risk of death. And those who expended up to 3,500 calories a week on exercise had a 54 percent improvement in longevity.

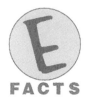

FACTS

According to experts, your calorie burn remains elevated for at least 30 minutes after vigorous exercise. This means you're still burning calories even if you're just watching television.

From this study, it's easy to assume that the more intense your exercise regimen, the longer you're likely to live. However, such is not the case. Dr. Paffenbarger's study found that men who expended more than 3,500 calories a week through exercise actually had a slightly smaller improvement in longevity than those who exercised more moderately.

Another study of male Harvard graduates compared longevity rates of major athletes (meaning those who lettered in a particular sport), minor athletes (those who participated but didn't letter), and nonathletes. It was assumed that the major athletes, who presumably exercised the hardest, would have the greatest longevity, but, in fact, it was the minor athletes who lived the longest.

What does this mean? Well, for starters, it means that when it comes to life-extending physical activity, moderation is best. There's no need to train like an Olympic athlete, because too much exercise is just as bad as too little. The key is to strengthen and maintain your body's systems, not abuse them, which is what an excessive physical regimen does. If you feel pain, you're working too hard. Slow down and listen to your body. It will tell you what it needs and when you've gone too far.

A Patron Saint of Exercise

Jack LaLanne is without a doubt the patron saint of physical fitness. Few people have helped promote the role of exercise and diet in longevity the way LaLanne has.

LaLanne is truly a self-made man. Born in 1914, he was a sickly child who developed into an underweight teenager with a serious sugar habit. His life changed, however, when he attended a lecture by Dr. Paul Bragg, a vocal proponent of the natural health movement. From that moment on, LaLanne devoted his life to developing his body through exercise and proper nutrition—and to helping others do the same.

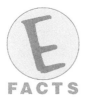

FACTS

A startling 54 percent of American adults are overweight. However, doctors diagnose obesity in only 38 percent of their overweight patients, and of those, only 25 percent receive advice from their doctors on weight loss, exercise, and diet.

In 1936, LaLanne opened the first commercial health club in Oakland, California. And, in doing so, he became the first person to actively promote weight training for women. In addition, he invented weight machines for specific sections of the body.

LaLanne's astounding physical feats have generated a lot of publicity over the years, for both himself and his workout regimen. Among the most remarkable are the following:

- At the age of sixty, LaLanne swam from Alcatraz Island to Fisherman's Wharf while handcuffed, shackled, and towing a 1,000-pound boat. When asked why, he quipped: "To give the prisoners hope."
- At age sixty-one, LaLanne celebrated the nation's bicentennial by swimming the length of Long Beach Harbor (about 1 mile) while handcuffed, shackled, and towing thirteen boats (one for each of the original thirteen colonies).
- At age sixty-two, LaLanne swam the length of the Golden Gate Bridge underwater while towing a 2,000-pound boat.
- At age sixty-five, LaLanne swam Japan's Lake Ashinoko while handcuffed, shackled, and towing sixty-five boats containing a total of 6,500 pounds of wood pulp.
- On his seventieth birthday, LaLanne braved strong currents and blustery winds to tow seventy boats and seventy people a total of 1.5 miles—again while handcuffed and shackled.

What's the secret to LaLanne's astounding physical endurance? The answer is, an astounding devotion to proper nutrition and rigorous exercise. He consumes about 450 vitamin and mineral supplements daily and eats nothing but natural foods. His diet is rich in fruits and vegetables, and he avoids red meat, substituting poultry instead. He also avoids dietary fat.

His exercise regimen is just as demanding. He works out two and a half hours each day, combining weight training with aerobic exercise for endurance.

Selecting the Fitness Club That's Right for You

For many people, the social atmosphere of a fitness club is ideal motivation for maintaining their workout regimen. In addition to featuring a huge array of exercise machines and free weights, many fitness clubs also offer individual instruction and other services, including step aerobic classes, yoga, and consultation with a nutrition or fitness expert. Care should be taken in selecting a gym or fitness club, because some are better than others. Here are a few tips:

- *Select a club that is close to home or work.* Convenience is an important factor in maintaining a regular fitness regimen; if you have to travel too far, you probably won't stick with it for very long.
- *Try it out before joining.* Most fitness clubs will allow you to work out at least once or twice before laying down your money (if the one you've chosen won't, go somewhere else). A couple of demo sessions lets you check out the equipment, the personnel, and the atmosphere.
- *Take a close look at the equipment.* Is it new and in good condition or old and worn? Is everything operational, or is half the equipment awaiting repair? A good club maintains its equipment and fixes problems quickly.
- *Visit the club during the times you are most likely to work out.* Most people visit the gym in the morning before work or in the evening after work. Is the facility so crowded during those times that

you have to wait forever to use a piece of equipment? If so, think twice before joining.

- *Find out how well trained the staff is and whether there is always someone on the floor to answer questions and help you with your workout.* A good health club will always have trained staff readily available.

- *Ask about classes.* A growing number of fitness clubs offer a wide variety of health and fitness services other than just use of the workout equipment. If these classes interest you, talk with the instructors regarding their training as well as class availability. Some clubs charge an additional fee for certain classes, such as yoga and fitness boxing.

- *Inquire about membership discounts.* Many clubs offer a variety of discounts or low-cost memberships, but often you have to inquire to receive them. Read the membership contract thoroughly and make sure you understand all provisions and requirements.

- *Make sure you feel comfortable.* Is the staff courteous and accommodating or too busy with their own workout to assist you? A good gym will go out of its way to make you feel at home.

- *Consider less expensive alternatives.* Fancy fitness clubs aren't for everyone; some people feel more at home in an old-fashioned gym, which often costs less. Call your local YMCA or municipal activities department for a list of low-cost workout facilities in your area.

Exercise Tips for Individual Populations

Regular exercise, to paraphrase those old milk commercials, is good for everybody, whether you're male, female, old, young, or differently abled. As noted throughout this book, the healthful benefits of exercise are many, and researchers are discovering new and different reasons to exercise every day.

But no single physical activity or exercise approach is right for all populations; the needs and abilities of men are different from those of women, just as the needs and abilities of younger people are different from those in their senior years. The goals of regular exercise are also as varied as the individuals who engage in it. Some people exercise to lose weight; others want to increase muscle mass, strength, or endurance. Whatever your personal goal may be, the key to success is perseverance. It may take some trial and error before you find the most satisfying and effective exercise regimen for your individual needs and abilities, but it's well worth it. As any doctor will tell you, exercise is one of the key components to adding many more healthful years to your life.

Exercise Tips for Men

Many men go through life with the erroneous belief that they don't need a regular exercise regimen. If you ask them why, they'll tell you they get sufficient exercise working in the yard on weekends, tossing the football with Junior before dinner, or playing a round of golf every other Saturday.

Those are all fine activities, but they are hardly sufficient to give the body the physical workout it needs to stay strong and healthy, and thus promote longevity. While studies show that an increasing number of men are joining fitness centers or team-sports activities in an attempt to stay physically fit, the sad fact is that many, many more need to get off the couch and onto the tennis court, cycling course, or baseball diamond.

If you're one of those men who is lacking the motivation to get out and exercise on a regular basis, now's the time to take action. It's never too late to improve your physical and mental health with a vigorous workout. Following are some helpful tips:

- *See a doctor before you begin your regimen.* This is especially important if you've been living a relatively sedentary lifestyle for several years, are noticeably overweight, or have a family history of heart disease or any other disorder that could be worsened by sudden physical exertion.
- *Don't try to be Mr. Macho.* Many men think they can go from Couch Potato to Carl Lewis in a single workout and end up injuring themselves in the process. The truth is that a lean, fit body isn't something you can achieve overnight; it takes time and dedication. So start slowly and gradually add to your workout.
- *Set realistic goals.* Do you want to lose 20 pounds? Run a marathon? Bench-press 250 pounds? Big jobs are always easier when broken

down into a series of smaller tasks. For example, if serious weight loss is your ultimate goal, vow to lose 5 pounds in your first month, then another 5 the next month. Before you know it, you'll have reached your goal of 20 pounds.

- *Vary your activities to ensure a complete workout.* Weight lifting strengthens your muscles; you'll also need some cardiovascular activity, such as aerobics, to benefit your heart and lungs.

- *Consult a personal trainer.* If you have trouble staying motivated, a personal trainer can be extremely beneficial. In addition to making sure you exercise regularly, he or she can show you how to perform your workout for maximum advantage.

- *Consider team sports.* Many are turned off by the regimented workout received at a fitness center. If you prefer company with your activity, consider joining a baseball, softball, tennis, or racquetball league. All of these activities benefit the heart, lungs, and muscles.

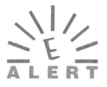

Remember: "No pain, no gain" is a myth. If you start to experience discomfort, end your session immediately. Pain could mean you're pushing yourself too hard or not performing an exercise properly. If pain lingers for more than three days, consult your doctor.

Exercise Tips for Women

Everyone needs regular exercise, but women need it for different reasons than men. In addition to improving cardiovascular function, exercise—particularly weight-bearing exercise—can go a long way toward preventing the onset of bone-destroying osteoporosis.

Exercise is also an important part of weight control (along with watching your caloric intake). Many women spend big bucks trying to slim down via fad diets, when all they really need to do is walk around the block every day or take an aerobics class at their local fitness center. Without question, exercise is the most effective and least expensive form of weight management available.

Following are some important tips to help women exercise properly and safely:

- *Engage in a variety of different exercises.* A well-rounded exercise regimen should strengthen muscles, benefit the heart and lungs, and build endurance. For optimum results, alternate weight training, aerobics, and circuit training. Reliance on only one form of exercise will not benefit your entire body.
- *Start slowly and work your way up.* It's natural to want to reach your maximum capacity as quickly as possible, but you have to be realistic; a gradual increase in weight or repetitions is the safest way to go. This is particularly true if you live a relatively sedentary lifestyle and are just beginning a serious exercise regimen.
- *Always warm up for five to ten minutes before engaging in strenuous exercise, and always cool down afterward.*
- *Drink plenty of fluids before, during, and after you exercise.* This keeps your body functioning at full capacity and prevents dehydration.
- *Maintain a safe pace.* Here's a good rule of thumb: If you can't speak while exercising, you need to slow down.

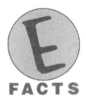

FACTS

Women who "yo-yo" diet (repeatedly lose weight, then gain it back) have significantly lower levels of so-called "good" cholesterol than women who maintain a steady weight, putting the dieters at increased risk of death from heart disease.

- *Consider using a personal trainer.* Most gyms have staff that will create the exercise regimen that's best for you and help you through it. This ensures that you are exercising correctly and at the proper pace. Having a personal trainer is also a good way to stay motivated.
- *Set a reasonable goal and reward yourself when you reach it.* For example, you might want to lose, say, 15 pounds or go down two dress sizes. Set a realistic date to achieve that goal, work toward it, and indulge yourself when you succeed. If you don't reach your goal by the set date, don't despair; re-evaluate your exercise regimen, set another target date, and go for it.
- *Consider some fun alternatives to the traditional exercise activities, such as calisthenics, dance aerobics, and yoga.* It's important that

you enjoy your exercise regimen, because it reduces the chances that you'll get bored and quit.

Exercise Tips for Seniors

As we grow older, it's common for us to slow down. Joints ache, bones weaken, systems slow. As a result, exercise becomes a thing of the past for many senior citizens. And this is a shame, because numerous studies support the beneficial effects of exercise on strength and aerobic power in older adults.

There can be other benefits to an active lifestyle as well. For example, some studies have shown that exercise may improve gait, balance, and physical function in older men and women. In addition, a training program can normalize glucose intolerance in elderly people and enhance the muscle's sensitivity to insulin. And the more physically active an older person is, the more calories he or she can consume without gaining unwanted pounds. For many, this parlays into better overall nutrition.

There's more: Regular exercise can promote bone density and thus reduce the risk of fractures—a common problem among the elderly. It is also believed that regular physical activity can lower the rate of functional decline in the elderly and possibly even improve neurological function, including memory.

Studies comparing seniors who exercise to those who don't found some striking differences between the two populations. For example, the exercisers typically were more aware of current health issues and had a more positive outlook regarding their own health. In addition, the exercisers were less likely to report having hypertension, arthritis, and other age-related ailments. Even in our senior years, it seems, exercise can slow the aging process!

While many seniors are physically unable to join a gym (though a sizable percentage of gym rats are sixty-five years and older), that doesn't mean older men and women can't exercise. Physical activity can take many forms, even for those with limited mobility. For example, walk around the house if you can't walk around the block. Putter in your garden. Lift light weights while watching television. The point is, do *something*.

Is it really worth it? Absolutely! Data from the Established Populations for Epidemiologic Studies of the Elderly revealed that after three years of study, the mortality of men and women who were moderately or highly active was $\frac{1}{2}$ to $\frac{2}{3}$ the mortality of those who never exercised.

Exercise Tips for the Differently Abled

Individuals living with a physical disability or chronic health problem often avoid regular exercise in the mistaken belief that they can't or shouldn't engage in strenuous physical activity. This may be true for certain conditions, but even heart patients can benefit from exercise when it's performed carefully and under a doctor's supervision.

Indeed, the physical and mental good of exercise should never be underestimated. For the differently abled, regular physical activity can keep limbs strong and limber; improve overall muscle tone; aid the heart, lungs, and other organs; and improve mood and mental function.

Following are some general tips on how to exercise safely and effectively:

- *Consult your doctor first.* This is an absolute must for anyone who lives with a physical disability or chronic health condition— no matter how minor. Before engaging in any strenuous exercise, see your doctor to make sure that your program won't worsen your condition or exacerbate a hidden medical disorder. Follow your doctor's advice and keep him or her apprised of any changes in your physical health.
- *Be aware of your physical limitations.* Start your exercise regimen slowly, never push yourself to exhaustion, and stop at the first indication of pain or injury.
- *Consider exercising in water.* Working out in the shallow end of a pool provides great exercise with minimal risk of strain or injury. The buoyancy provided by a pool regimen can be especially beneficial to individuals who have limited use of their limbs.
- *Exercise with supervision.* The need for supervision depends on the type and extent of your condition or disability. Not everyone will need it, but if there is even a slight possibility that you could be injured

while exercising, try to work out with a friend, relative, or professional trainer, just to be safe.

ESSENTIALS

If you ask fifty doctors, they'll all tell you the following: The most effective way to lose weight is to eat with nutrition in mind and to exercise more. But that doesn't stop Americans from spending millions of dollars on fad diets and other weight-loss gimmicks each year. The Food and Nutrition Science Alliance offers these tips for identifying dangerous fad diets:

- It sounds too good to be true.
- It offers a quick fix and requires little effort.
- It focuses almost exclusively on a particular food or food group.
- It derives simplistic conclusions from complicated studies or is based on only one study.
- Its claims have been repeatedly disputed by reputable nutrition experts.

The Role of Nutrition

Now that we've got the exercise thing figured out, let's move on to our next favorite subject: nutrition. It's possible to eat junk food our whole lives and still live to be 120; it's just not very likely. Nutrition, perhaps more than any other factor, plays an essential role in our overall health and longevity.

The reason for this is simple: The foods we eat affect virtually every cell, organ, and system in our bodies. If we eat enough of the right foods, our bodies thrive, and we live well and long. If we insist on stuffing ourselves with the wrong kinds of foods, our bodies suffer, placing us at increased risk of disease and, ultimately, limiting our longevity.

The role of nutrition can't be overstated. According to nutrition experts, a healthful diet provides our cells with everything they need to function well, reproduce, and repair damage from a variety of sources. Healthful foods also give our bodies the right kind of fuel so that we have plenty of energy and a strong immune system.

But there's more. The right kinds of foods help our bodies get rid of waste products and potentially harmful toxins, many of which can increase our risk of serious illness, including cancer, if not purged regularly. And they help reduce our risk of many chronic disorders commonly associated with aging, including osteoporosis and heart disease.

Unfortunately, too many people—children included—eat without considering their health. Home meals are prepared with convenience rather than nutrition in mind or are too often replaced by fat- and sodium-laden fast food. Processed foods replace whole foods, and sweet, sugary desserts are given more attention than the main course. All of this wreaks havoc with our health and well-being, though very often we're blind to these effects.

But the fact remains: If you want to live a long time and enjoy those extra years, you have to eat well. This doesn't mean eating like a monk or giving up your favorite foods. It doesn't even mean giving up your favorite desserts! It simply means eating in moderation, eating less of those foods that may not be the best for us (such as overly processed foods, fried foods, and fatty slabs of red meat), and placing a greater emphasis on foods known for their high nutrition. Fortunately, it's a lot easier than it sounds.

Good Foods/Bad Foods

When we're hungry, any food is good food. A growling belly is satisfied by just about anything, whether it's steamed broccoli or a bag of pork rinds. But not all foods are created equal; some are good for us, and some are bad for us. And some can be good or bad, depending on how much we consume and in what form.

It's interesting to note that the concept of what's good for us has changed dramatically over the years. It used to be that a so-called "complete meal" meant plenty of red meat and dairy, with some veggies on the side. Now we know that red meat, while still a source of nutrition, is best consumed in smaller quantities and with as much fat removed as possible. In recent decades, the dietary value of fruits and vegetables has become increasingly evident, to the point where they are now the mainstay of a healthy diet, along with poultry, fish, whole grain breads, and legumes. Perhaps ten years from now, the Nutrition Pyramid will change again as more information is uncovered regarding the foods we eat and the nutrition they provide.

It's sometimes difficult to categorize foods as "bad" and "good" because there can be quite a bit of crossover. A steak now and then is a good source of protein as well as other nutrients, but eating steak four days a week is just asking for a heart attack. Likewise, fruit and vegetables are a wonderful source of essential nutrients (many of which, such as antioxidants, can help slow the aging process), but a strict vegetarian diet can lead to malnutrition if not adequately balanced and supplemented.

In general, however, fried foods should be consumed in moderation. Sugar consumption should also be limited, though that's very hard to do in the traditional American diet. Nonetheless, it's well worth the effort. Alcohol, too, should be consumed in moderation, perhaps a maximum of one or two glasses a day. Alcohol is considered a neurotoxin, and more than two glasses a day can adversely affect your health.

The list of good foods is far longer than the list of bad foods and includes fruits and vegetables, legumes, whole grain products, pasta, poultry, and fish. If these items are the mainstay of your diet, except for the occasional steak or hot fudge sundae, you're well on the way to a long life.

Dietary Guidelines from the American Heart Association

- Dietary fat intake should be less than 30 percent of total calories.
- Saturated fat intake should be less than 10 percent of total calories.
- Polyunsaturated fat should not exceed 10 percent of total calories.
- Cholesterol intake should not exceed 300 milligrams per day.
- Carbohydrate intake should represent 50 percent or more total calories with emphasis on complex carbohydrates.
- Protein intake should constitute the remainder of the calories.
- Sodium intake should be limited to less than 3 grams per day.
- Alcohol consumption is not recommended, but if consumed, it should not exceed 1 ounce a day of hard liquor, 8 ounces of wine, or 24 ounces of beer.

Phytonutrients

Phyto is the Greek word for plant; phytonutrients are the vitamins and minerals derived from fruits and vegetables. In nature, phytonutrients protect plants from natural predators such as insects and bacteria, and when we eat plants, these same chemicals protect us as well. The health problems prevented by the phytonutrients we consume every day include everything from elevated cholesterol and heart disease to cancer and even aging. Think of them as nature's pharmacy—free, safe, and readily available.

Some of the most important phytonutrients, according to nutrition experts, include the following:

- *Allylic sulfides.* These compounds give onions, garlic, and related herbs their pungent odor and unique flavor and have a long history as important nutrients. Their benefits are many, including raising HDL cholesterol (the so-called "good cholesterol"), lowering blood triglyceride levels, protecting the heart, and stimulating the production of enzymes believed to suppress the growth of certain types of tumors.
- *Carotenoids.* These compounds are found in abundance in carrots, broccoli, cantaloupe, cauliflower, green leafy vegetables, and tomatoes. They are powerful antioxidants and play an instrumental role in preventing heart disease and certain forms of cancer.
- *Flavonoids.* Also members of the antioxidant family, these chemicals can be found in apples, citrus fruit, cranberries, endive, grape juice, kale, onions, and red wine. Their primary benefit is the prevention of heart disease and blood clots.
- *Indoles and isothiocyanates.* These compounds are plentiful in broccoli, cabbage, cauliflower, and mustard greens. They help stimulate enzymes known to prevent cancer and block estrogen activity in cells.
- *Isoflavones.* These chemicals, which also prevent the formation of certain cancers and block estrogen activity in the cells, can be found in chickpeas, kidney beans, lentils, and soybeans.
- *Lignans.* These chemicals are known antioxidants and block estrogen activity in the cells as well as help prevent the formation of certain cancers. They are particularly abundant in flaxseed.

- *Monoterpenes.* Yet another cancer preventative, this phytonutrient blocks the action of certain cancer-causing compounds. It can be found in citrus fruits such as oranges and grapefruit, as well as cherries.
- *Phenolic compounds.* These antioxidants help activate important cancer-fighting enzymes. To add them to your diet, eat plenty of fruit, vegetables, and cereal grains, and drink green or black teas.
- *Saponins.* These chemicals bind with cholesterol and help the body flush it out. They also stimulate the immune system and help prevent heart disease and certain types of cancer. They can be found in chickpeas, nuts, oats, potatoes, soybeans, spinach, and tomatoes.

What Phytonutrients Can Do for You

As already noted, phytonutrients help protect us in three specific ways: They flush toxic chemicals from our bodies, inhibit free radical damage, and keep certain hormones, such as estrogen, at optimal levels.

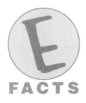
FACTS

The French are living examples of the benefits of phytonutrients. Even though their diet is packed with rich dishes, they smoke a lot, and they drink a sea of red wine, their rate of heart disease is nearly 2½ times less than that of Americans. The French diet is also loaded with fresh fruits and vegetables—items rich in flavonoids. According to several clinical studies, flavonoids help keep cholesterol from sticking to artery walls. This, in turn, helps prevent arterial blockages and heart disease. Aiding the French even more is the fact that red wine is also packed with flavonoids—an added bonus.

This third mechanism is especially important for women. Estrogen is a valuable hormone necessary for the regulation of many functions, including menstruation and childbirth. It also plays an integral role in the prevention of heart disease by keeping cholesterol levels under control. However, estrogen also has its bad side. When levels get above a certain point, the hormone can stimulate hormone-related cancers, including breast and ovarian cancer. Isoflavones and similar phytonutrients, which act very much like natural estrogen, prevent this from happening by binding with estrogen receptors. As a result, the extra estrogen produced by the body has nothing to bind to and is flushed out.

Of course, hormone-stimulated cancers aren't the only ones affected by phytonutrients. Recent studies have uncovered a wide array of benefits from the fruits and vegetables most commonly included in the traditional American diet. Carrots and green leafy vegetables, for example, appear to reduce risk of lung cancer. And cruciferous vegetables—particularly broccoli and cauliflower—have been shown to reduce the risk of colon cancer.

Vitamins and Minerals

The foods that make up a healthy diet contain a wide variety of vitamins and minerals. Some are more involved in slowing the aging process than others, but all play a role in our overall health. We don't have room to examine every single vitamin and mineral necessary for perfect health, but the following advice and information should be included in everyone's anti-aging regimen.

Vitamins

"Take your vitamins or you'll get sick!" How many times did you hear that as a child growing up? If you're like most people, it was probably one of your mother's favorite refrains. But she was right; vitamins are vital to our health and longevity.

Vitamins—complex molecules that keep the body's chemical mechanisms functioning properly—come in a wide variety and perform a huge number of jobs. Every vitamin has a specific task or benefit that is unique in and of itself. Therefore, as you plan out your anti-aging diet, it's important that you know what each type of vitamin is and how it can benefit you.

Vitamin A

Also known as retinol, vitamin A is a fat-soluble vitamin that helps regulate cell development, promotes bone and tooth development, and boosts the body's immune system. In addition, by helping to form rhodopsin, a substance needed by the eyes to function in partial darkness, vitamin A helps us see at night. Vitamin A is available in two forms: as vitamin A and as beta-carotene, a plant-based compound that the body converts into vitamin A. Plentiful sources include apricots, broccoli, cantaloupe, carrots, lettuce, liver, and sweet potatoes. The RDA for vitamin A is 5,000 international units for men and 4,000 international units for women. Women who are pregnant or breastfeeding should take an additional 1,000 international units daily.

Vitamin B_2

More commonly known as riboflavin, vitamin B_2 plays an important role during growth and development. It keeps the mucous membranes healthy; helps protect the nervous system, eyes, and skin; and boosts iron absorption. Interestingly, vitamin B_2 is commonly used in the treatment of a wide assortment of medical problems, including infections and burns. Good sources for the vitamin include milk, cheese, yogurt, chicken, green leafy vegetables, and bread. The RDA for vitamin B_2 is 1.6 milligrams for men aged twenty-three to fifty, 1.4 milligrams for men fifty-one and older, 1.3 milligrams for women up to age twenty-two, and 1.2 milligrams for women twenty-three and older. Pregnant women require an additional 0.3 milligrams daily, and women who are breastfeeding require an extra 0.5 milligrams.

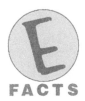

FACTS

Government health experts report that nearly a third of Americans—approximately 58 million—are clinically obese, which is defined as 20 percent over their ideal weight.

Vitamin B_3

More commonly known as niacin, vitamin B_3 is instrumental in maintaining the health of the skin, nerves, and digestive system. It also helps release energy from the food we eat, aids in the synthesis of DNA, and helps lower blood levels of cholesterol and triglycerides, because of the nicotinic acid form of the vitamin. Dietary sources of vitamin B_3 include lean meats, fish, poultry, peanuts, brewer's yeast, and sunflower seeds. The RDA for vitamin B_3 is 18 milligrams for men age twenty-three to fifty, 16 milligrams for men fifty and older, 14 milligrams for women fifteen to twenty-two, and 13 milligrams for women twenty-three and older. Pregnant women require an extra 2 milligrams of vitamin B_3 during pregnancy and an additional 4 milligrams while breastfeeding.

Vitamin B_6

Also known as pyridoxine and pyridoxal, vitamin B_6 plays a very important role in maintaining the body's immune system. It also helps the brain work properly, enables the body to resist stress, helps maintain the proper chemical balance in the body's fluids, works with other vitamins and minerals to supply the energy used by muscles, and is influential in cell growth. Sources include avocados, bananas, carrots, fish, lentils, meat, rice, soybeans, and whole grains. The RDA for vitamin B_6 is 2.2 milligrams for men and 2.0 milligrams for women. Pregnant women need an additional 0.6 milligrams each day, and breastfeeding women need an extra 0.5 milligrams daily.

Vitamin B_{12}

This water-soluble vitamin is found in meat, fish, and dairy products, but not in fruits or vegetables. As a result, people on a strict vegetarian diet may develop a B_{12} deficiency if they don't take a vitamin supplement. Vitamin B_{12} enables the body to process carbohydrates and fats. It also helps the nervous system function properly and assists in growth and cell development, particularly blood cells. Vitamin B_{12} is also needed for the creation of the protective sheath that covers nerve cells and helps the body process DNA. The RDA for vitamin B_{12} is 3 micrograms for both men and women. Pregnant and breastfeeding women need an extra microgram of the vitamin daily.

Vitamin C

This vitamin, also known as ascorbic acid, is an important antioxidant and as such protects the body from free radicals, as well as helps repair damaged tissue. Vitamin C is also necessary for the manufacture of collagen (the connective tissue that holds bones together), helps with the absorption of iron, assists with the production of hemoglobin and red blood cells, keeps the gums and teeth healthy, and helps with wound healing. Dietary sources of vitamin C include citrus and other types of fruit, broccoli, brussels sprouts, green peppers, spinach, and tomatoes. The RDA for vitamin C is 60 milligrams for both men and women. Women who are pregnant require an additional 20 milligrams each day, and women who are breastfeeding should get an extra 40 milligrams daily.

Vitamin D

This vitamin comes in two forms: ergocalciferol (which is found in a small number of foods) and cholecalciferol (which the body manufactures when exposed to sunlight). It is required for the normal growth and development of teeth, bones, and connective tissue in children, as well as bone and tooth maintenance in adults. A vitamin D deficiency can result in rickets, which is characterized by brittle bones in adults. Dietary sources of vitamin D include fortified milk, herring, salmon, and sardines. The RDA for vitamin D is 600 international units for adults nineteen to twenty-two years and 400 international units for adults twenty-three and older. Women who are pregnant or breastfeeding require an additional 400 international units of vitamin D daily.

Vitamin E

This vitamin, like vitamin C, is a powerful antioxidant and helps protect cell membranes from damaging free radicals. It also assists in the production of red blood cells, helps prevent blood clots, and is believed to reduce development of certain types of cancer. Dietary sources of vitamin E include almonds, hazelnuts, sunflower seeds, walnuts, wheat germ, and various fruits and vegetables, including apples, blackberries, lettuce, onions, pears, and spinach. The RDA for vitamin E is 30 international units for men and 24 international units for women. Women who are pregnant need an additional 6 international units daily, and women who are breastfeeding require an extra 9 international units each day.

Minerals

When discussing nutrition, minerals are often mentioned in the same breath as vitamins. They serve a similar purpose in maintaining proper cell, organ, and system function and often work hand in hand with specific vitamins. Some minerals are more important than others to our overall health. We'll go through a few of the more important minerals together and take a look at exactly how they can benefit your longevity.

Calcium

Calcium is the most plentiful mineral in the body. This essential mineral works with phosphorus to maintain our bones and teeth. When our daily intake of calcium is too low, osteoporosis and other problems can result. Calcium also plays a role in the transmission of nerve impulses, promotes blood coagulation, and enables muscles, particularly the heart, to relax and contract. Dietary sources of calcium include dairy products, shrimp, canned fish such as salmon and sardines, green leafy vegetables, soybeans, and yogurt. The RDA for calcium is 800 milligrams for all adults, though many experts believe more is better. Women who are pregnant or breastfeeding need an extra 400 milligrams daily. Postmenopausal women are generally advised to consume 1,500 milligrams of calcium daily.

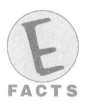

FACTS

Wine lovers may have a new reason to toast their favorite drink. New research suggests that wine drinkers live longer than those who drink beer and liquor. Wine seems to have a protective effect beyond that of just alcohol. Light drinkers who consumed one to seven drinks per week had a lower risk of death from heart disease or cancer, but the risk was reduced even further for light or moderate drinkers who consumed mostly wine.

Iron

This mineral is an important component of hemoglobin, the part of red blood cells that carries oxygen throughout the body. In fact, hemoglobin stores an estimated 70 percent of the body's iron supply; the remaining 30 percent is stored in muscle tissue and helps deliver the oxygen needed to make the muscles contract. An iron deficiency can result in anemia, characterized by an inability to get sufficient blood oxygen to cells. Dietary sources of iron include cheddar cheese, chickpeas, enriched bread, lentils, nuts, prune juice, and wheat germ. The RDA for iron is 10 milligrams for men nineteen and older, 18 milligrams for women eleven to fifty, and 10 milligrams for women fifty-one and older. Women who are pregnant or breastfeeding require an additional 50 milligrams of iron daily, though pregnant women should not take iron supplements during the first trimester of pregnancy unless prescribed by their physician.

Magnesium

This mineral is instrumental in a lot of different body functions, including the absorption of calcium and moving sodium and potassium across cell membranes. Magnesium also helps nerve impulses travel through the body, helps maintain the body's metabolism, and aids muscle function—including that of the heart. Magnesium can be obtained from many types of fish, fruits, green leafy vegetables, dairy products, nuts, and wheat germ. The RDA for magnesium is 350 milligrams for men and 300 milligrams for women. Women who are pregnant or breastfeeding should take an extra 150 milligrams of magnesium daily, preferably from dietary sources. Doctors recommend against taking magnesium supplements during pregnancy.

Phosphorus

The second most plentiful mineral in the human body is phosphorus. Phosphorus is important in maintaining healthy bones and teeth. It also plays a role in all chemical reactions in the body, helps the body metabolize several B vitamins, aids in the healing of fractures, helps the body produce energy, and boosts the growth, maintenance, and repair of all types of tissue. Plentiful sources of phosphorus include red meat and calves liver, poultry, fish, dairy products, peanuts, dried beans, peas, soybeans, and whole grains. The RDA for phosphorus is 800 milligrams for all adults. Women who are pregnant or breastfeeding should get an additional 400 milligrams of phosphorus daily.

Potassium

This is one of the most important minerals in the maintenance of healthy body function. Among other things, potassium keeps the heart beating normally, helps muscles contract, and feeds cells by controlling the transfer of nutrients from surrounding fluids. Potassium also helps the kidneys remove waste products from the body, helps provide oxygen to the brain, and works with calcium to regulate nerve function. The best dietary sources of potassium include avocados, bananas, citrus fruit, milk, nuts, potatoes, spinach, tomatoes, and whole grains. There is no standard RDA for potassium because requirements are affected by the amount of salt you consume in your diet, though most nutrition experts believe 2,000 to 2,500 milligrams to be a good daily minimum. Since most people get sufficient potassium from their diet, supplements are required only if you are taking medications that deplete your natural potassium reserves.

Selenium

The primary function of selenium is to protect cells from damaging free radicals. Good sources of selenium include broccoli, cabbage, celery, chicken, garlic, liver, onions, and whole grains. There is no established RDA for selenium, though men and women can safely consume between 50 and 200 micrograms daily.

Zinc

This trace element is part of the molecular structure of dozens of important enzymes, is a component of the insulin that regulates our energy supply, and works with red blood cells to transport waste carbon dioxide from body tissue to the lungs, where it is expelled. Zinc is also vital to the production of the RNA and DNA that oversees the division, growth, and repair of the body's cells; helps preserve our sense of taste and smell; and aids in wound healing. Dietary sources of zinc include beef, herring, pork, poultry, milk, soybeans, and whole grains. The RDA for zinc is 15 milligrams. Women who are pregnant should take an additional 5 milligrams of zinc daily, and women who are breastfeeding should take an extra 10 milligrams.

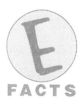

FACTS

The elimination of dead skin cells is a never-ending process. Over the course of our lives, we shed about 40 pounds of skin. In fact, a large percentage of house dust is actually discarded skin cells— a favorite food of microscopic mites.

The Importance of Fiber

Fiber has received a huge amount of publicity in recent years for its many health benefits, not the least of which is the possible prevention of certain types of cancer. As a result of this press and encouragement from physicians, people are working harder than ever to add more fiber to their diet, even if it's just an extra bran muffin at breakfast. In doing so, they may be adding many extra years to their lives.

The whole fiber phenomenon started in the 1970s, when researchers noticed that certain groups in Africa appeared to have a lower incidence of colon cancer as a result of their high fiber consumption. Later studies also found an association between high fiber intake and reduced rates of breast cancer. However, it's important to note that fiber alone may not be responsible for these benefits. Many diets high in fiber are also low in fat, and this could play an important role in reducing cancer risk. Nonetheless, fiber is an important part of a nutritionally sound diet, and you should do all you can to make sure you are getting sufficient amounts.

But what is fiber? Nutritionally speaking, it's the indigestible part of the food we eat—the stuff that passes through our digestive system relatively quickly and intact, such as the bran in grain, the pulp in fruit, and the skin of certain vegetables such as corn. The speed with which fiber travels through our digestive system is what makes it so healthful. By traveling so quickly, it also rushes other foods through our system, giving cancer-causing compounds less time to do their dirty work. It is also believed that fiber dilutes potential carcinogens, reducing their ability to do harm. And fiber also promotes healthy digestion by stimulating the action of beneficial bacteria.

There are four major types of fiber:

- *Cellulose.* This is the most common type of fiber and is found in most fruits and vegetables, as well as whole grains and some types of nuts. Cellulose is an effective stool softener and helps dilute bile acids in the colon, which are believed to stimulate the growth of certain types of cancer.

- *Gums.* These are sticky fibers derived from plants. They help lower cholesterol and prevent certain types of cancer, though researchers are still trying to figure out exactly how they work. Gums are found in oat bran, dried beans, and oatmeal and are commonly used to thicken processed foods.
- *Lignin.* This fiber acts as a binder for cellulose and is found in certain fruits, nuts, peas, tomatoes, and whole grains. It doesn't have the same action as cellulose on stools or bile acids, but laboratory studies have shown that it can help prevent the onset of cancer.
- *Pectin.* This gelatinous compound supplements the action of cellulose. It helps limit the potential damage from bile acids and also aids digestion by preventing diarrhea. Rich sources of pectin include apples, bananas, beets, carrots, and a wide array of citrus fruit.

Are you getting enough fiber in your diet? Probably not. Despite efforts by government health agencies to boost fiber intake, the typical American still consumes an average of only 11 grams a day. According to the National Cancer Institute, an amount double that would be far more healthful. Studies have shown that consuming between 20 and 30 grams of fiber a day can dramatically reduce your risk of many cancers. Consuming more than that, however, can cause painful and embarrassing bloating and flatulence. To avoid these problems, you should introduce fiber into your diet gradually and try to get as much as you can from the foods you eat, rather than relying on fiber supplements.

The Fat Problem

One of the most problematic foods in the typical American diet is fat. Our bodies need a certain amount of plant and animal fat to function well, but too much fat can lead to a whole host of medical problems ranging from heart disease to cancer to diabetes. Headlines about the hazards of fat have sent many people fleeing from the word, hell-bent on eliminating ALL fat from their diet. However, this is an impossibility, and it's also dangerous. Rather than a no-fat diet, we should be aiming for a low-fat diet. That way our bodies get what they need without increasing our risk of disease.

Dietary fats and oils, or triglycerides, are a source of energy and help produce compounds that regulate a variety of bodily functions, including blood clotting and blood pressure. They can be saturated or unsaturated, and unsaturated fats can be either monounsaturated or polyunsaturated. All triglycerides supply approximately 250 calories per ounce—more than double the calories supplied by equal amounts of protein or carbohydrates.

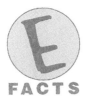
FACTS

Fish is much more than just "brain food." Regular consumption can also help protect your heart, reduce your risk of cancer, and slow the aging process. In a recent study at the University of Washington in Seattle, researchers found that a regular diet of fish helps prevent arteries from clogging and, more importantly, helps prevent cardiac arrest from irregular contractions of the heart. This is significant because cardiac arrest often strikes with no symptoms and is believed to result in nearly 250,000 deaths a year.

Saturated fats are "bad" because they tend to raise cholesterol levels and endanger the heart and other systems. These types of fat are usually solid at room temperature, such as the fat found in well-marbled meat. Major sources of saturated fats include butter, whole milk, cheese, ice cream, egg yolks, and fatty cuts of beef, pork, and lamb. Certain vegetable fats, such as palm, palm kernel, and coconut oils, are also saturated.

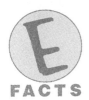
FACTS

Less than one-third of Americans meet the U.S. government's Healthy People 2000 goal of eating five or more servings (½ cup per serving) of fruits and vegetables a day. In fact, the majority of people eat only 1.2 servings of fruit and 3.1 servings of vegetables each day.

There are several ways to cut down on the amount of saturated fat in your diet. One is to make sure that all the meat you eat is as lean as possible, and that all excess fat has been trimmed away before you eat it. It also helps to replace the saturated fat in your diet with monounsaturated fats such as olive oil, peanut oil, canola oil, and certain fish oils. This can go a long way toward reducing both your blood cholesterol levels and your risk of heart disease.

Omega-3 fatty acids, or fish oils, can also help lower cholesterol and reduce your risk of disease. Effective sources include bluefish, herring, mackerel, rainbow trout, salmon, sardines, tuna, and whitefish.

Nutrition and Mental Acuity

The brain, like the body, is heavily influenced by the foods we eat. When we eat properly, brain function is strong; when we eat poorly, brain function is diminished. As we grow older, nutrition becomes even more important in maintaining mental acuity. We'll go through a quick review of some of the most important brain nutrients.

Amino Acids

Amino acids, simply put, are organic compounds that help make proteins and are essential to human metabolism. Though they don't receive nearly as much mention in nutrition discussions as vitamins and minerals, they are just as necessary to our health—particularly for brain function. Let's take a closer look at some of the most important amino acids in terms of maintaining mental acuity:

- *Arginine.* This amino acid is partially converted into a chemical known as spermine, which is believed to help the brain process memory. Because of this action, low levels of spermine often signal age-related memory loss.
- *Choline.* The brain uses this amino acid to manufacture a memory-related neurotransmitter called acetylcholine. Older people are encouraged to take choline supplements because as we age we tend to produce less acetylcholine, putting us at greater risk of memory impairment. Dietary sources of choline include cabbage, cauliflower, eggs, peanuts, and lecithin.
- *Glutamine.* This amino acid is a precursor of a calming neurotransmitter known as GABA. It also helps improve clarity of thought and boosts alertness by assisting in the manufacture of

glutamic acid, a compound known for its ability to eliminate metabolic wastes in the brain.

- *Methionine.* Like glutamine, this amino acid helps cleanse the brain of damaging metabolic wastes. It is an effective antioxidant and helps reduce brain levels of dangerous heavy metals such as mercury.

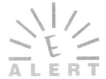

Most businesses have banned smoking, forcing smokers to take their habit outside for the comfort and safety of all. However, passive smoke is still a problem in this country and can result in some serious health issues, particularly among family members of smokers. A recent study examining the impact of passive smoking among police in Hong Kong was reported in the *Journal of Epidemiology and Community Health*.

The report's most important conclusion: Workers forced to breathe in their colleagues' cigarette smoke are significantly more likely to take sick leave and require medical attention.

Vitamins

Your brain needs just as many vitamins as the rest of your body does, and it gets them from the bloodstream. When vitamin absorption is reduced or impeded as a result of a poor diet or an illness, the brain is one of the first organs to feel it. We'll go through a quick rundown of some of the more essential vitamins needed for long-term brain health.

- *Vitamin A.* This antioxidant helps protect brain cells from harmful free radicals and benefits the circulatory system so blood flow to the brain remains strong.
- *Vitamin B_{12}.* An estimated 25 percent of people between ages sixty and seventy are deficient in this essential nutrient, as are nearly 40 percent of people eighty and older. A B_{12} deficiency may be mistaken for an age-related decline in mental function, including memory loss and a reduction in reasoning skills. To hedge your bet, take a multivitamin tablet daily.

- *Vitamin B$_6$.* This important vitamin helps convert sugar into glucose, which the brain needs for fuel. It also benefits general circulation, which can improve memory. Older people need substantially more B$_6$ than younger people, so make sure your diet is packed with this nutrient.
- *Vitamin B$_1$.* Like B$_{12}$, this nutrient is a potent antioxidant. It also is required for numerous metabolic processes within the brain and peripheral nervous system.
- *Folic acid.* This nutrient, also a member of the B vitamin family, is known to aid cerebral circulation by inhibiting narrowing of the arteries in the neck. Studies also suggest that daily supplements of folic acid can reduce the likelihood of certain age-related psychiatric problems, including dementia.
- *Vitamin C.* This well-known antioxidant is extremely important for proper brain function and, as such, is found in much higher levels within the brain than other parts of the body. In addition to boosting the effectiveness of other antioxidants, vitamin C is an essential ingredient in the manufacture of several neurotransmitters such as dopamine and acetylcholine. In short, a daily dose of vitamin C can boost and maintain mental acuity. So important is vitamin C to proper brain function that it is being evaluated as a possible nutritional preventative for Alzheimer's disease.
- *Vitamin E.* Yet another important antioxidant, vitamin E also restores damaged neurotransmitter receptor sites on neurons. This means that vitamin E both prevents age-related brain deterioration and also reverses a specific aspect of that breakdown. There is also evidence that vitamin E can prevent the onset of Alzheimer's disease and slow its progression once it develops, and that a combination of vitamin E and the mineral selenium can dramatically improve mood and cognitive function in older patients. In addition, vitamin E can help reduce risk of heart disease, stroke, and certain types of cancer.

Minerals

Like vitamins, a wide array of minerals are also extremely important in maintaining cognitive function throughout life. And as in the rest of the body, minerals often work hand in hand with vitamins in the brain to get the job done. Let's take a closer look at some of the most important minerals for preserving cognitive function.

- *Magnesium.* This mineral is an absolute must for proper brain function in that it aids neuron metabolism, helps reduce brain damage from ischemia (a lack of blood flow to the brain), and boosts the effectiveness of certain antioxidants. Magnesium may also play a role in the prevention of Alzheimer's disease, since studies show that the brains of most AD patients are magnesium deficient but excessively high in calcium. (In healthy brains, the two minerals have a relatively equal ratio.) In addition, magnesium improves circulation by inhibiting dangerous blood clots and reducing blood pressure.
- *Selenium.* This very powerful antioxidant benefits the brain by preventing oxidation of fat. Why is this important? It's important because more than half of the brain is composed of a type of fat. By inhibiting oxidation, selenium slows age-related brain deterioration and preserves cognitive function. Selenium also benefits the immune system, and some studies suggest that it improves circulation throughout the body. Because selenium levels tend to decline with age, older people should take selenium supplements in addition to adding selenium-rich foods to their diets.
- *Zinc.* This mineral aids the brain as part of a metabolic process that eliminates harmful free radicals. It also strengthens neuronal membranes for greater protection and helps get rid of lead, which can enter the brain through automobile exhaust and other sources and adversely affect mental function.

Selecting the Right Anti-aging Foods for You

Some foods are better for you than others. The key is to eat a diverse diet, with an emphasis on those foods known to pack the greatest nutritional punch.

Fruits and vegetables should be your biggest concern, because the majority of Americans don't consume nearly as much as they should. Government health officials suggest five servings of fruit and vegetables daily—which is twice the amount suggested for meat and dairy. Fruits and vegetables are an important part of any anti-aging regimen because they are packed with essential nutrients in their most natural and useful form.

Almost all fruits and vegetables are good for you, but some are better than others. When it comes to fruit, apples, bananas, berries, citrus fruit, and melons are your best bets because of their high fiber and nutrient content. As for vegetables, it's a good idea to load your diet with as many cruciferous vegetables as possible because of their cancer-preventing antioxidant properties (as well as other healthful benefits). The most potent cruciferous vegetables include bok choy (Chinese cabbage), broccoli, brussels sprouts, cabbage, cauliflower, collard greens, kale, mustard greens, rutabagas, turnips, and watercress. Also high in nutrition are carrots, celery, potatoes, spinach, sweet potatoes, and tomatoes (which contain a cancer-fighting compound known as lycopene).

Cereal grains should also be a big part of your daily diet. They provide much needed fiber as well as a variety of important vitamins and minerals.

Limit your consumption of red meat; the red meat you do eat should be as lean as possible. More healthful alternatives include poultry, legumes, and deep-water fish such as tuna, mackerel, herring, shrimp, and salmon, all of which contain nutritious omega-3 fatty acids.

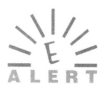

People afflicted with lactose intolerance—an inability to adequately digest dairy products—should consider taking calcium supplements to ensure that they're getting the recommended daily allowance.

Dairy products are a good source of calcium as well as other vitamins and minerals, but they should be low-fat if possible. People who are lactose intolerant should explore non-dairy alternatives and should consider taking calcium supplements to prevent age-related osteoporosis and similar disorders.

CHAPTER 4

Herbal Remedies

The use of herbs as both medicine and nutritional supplements has never been more popular. In fact, herbs are now used to treat or prevent conditions as diverse as depression and the common cold. Should herbs play a role in your anti-aging regimen? The answer is yes—but only if you use them moderately and intelligently. The fact is, herbs have a centuries-old history as medicinal compounds, and early studies seem to bear out that they do, indeed, work. Let's take a look at the use of herbal remedies in your anti-aging regimen.

Herbs and Your Anti-aging Regimen

Although the use of herbs for medicinal purposes is not a new concept, many people are unaware of how herbs can and will benefit their overall health. The whole idea of herbal remedies may open up a completely new approach towards anti-aging and maintaining a healthful lifestyle. Throughout this chapter, we're going to take a look at a variety of herbal remedies, as well as how they work and what they can do to increase your longevity.

Your Herbal Medicinal Choices

The word *herb,* as used in herbal remedies, is also known as "botanical medicine" and, in Europe, "phytotherapy" or "phytomedicine." All of these terms simply mean that a plant part is used to make a medicinal preparation. An herb can be the entire plant or any of its parts, which include the leaf, flower, stem, seed, root, fruit, and bark.

One way to categorize herbs is by looking at what kinds of ailment respond to their use. Another way is to look at how many of our modern-day drugs are based on herbal components. These synthesized substances, now known as drugs, have been separated out from the whole plant by various means.

One of the first modern drugs to be isolated from a plant was morphine, which was first identified in 1803 by the German Friedrich Seturner. Using opium poppy plants, he extracted white crystals from them using techniques that soon became routine. As a result, aconitine was made from monkshood, emetine from ipecacuanha, atropine from deadly nightshade, and quinine from Peruvian bark. All of these synthesized compounds, categorized as alkaloids, were extremely potent and previously could be obtained only from the raw plants themselves.

The original breakthrough of converting the actual plant into a "pill" came in 1852, when salicin, which had been identified as one of the active ingredients in willow bark, was artificially synthesized for the first time. Later, acetylsalicylic acid, what we now know as aspirin, was chemically modified because the product proved to upset the stomach lining in some people. In 1899, acetylsalicylic acid was launched into the marketplace by the Bayer drug company.

Since then, plant extracts have become commonplace on pharmacy shelves. Ephedrine preparations from *ma huang* are available both in over-the-counter and prescription form.

To date, out of the approximately 500,000 plant species on Earth, only about 5,000 have been thoroughly studied for their medicinal value. This means that there is still a vast number of plants that may hold hidden within their leaves, seeds, flowers, fruits, stem, barks, and roots the cures from some of humanity's most perplexing diseases, such as cancer, AIDS, diabetes, or other illnesses today considered incurable. This fact alone should make us treat all plant life, and especially herbal plant life, with great respect.

The Value of Plants in Health and Healing

In many parts of the world, herbs are the only option available to treat medical problems. Because herbs take an indirect route to the bloodstream, their effects are usually slower and more subtle that purified drugs administered by a doctor writing a prescription. In Colonial America and well into the nineteenth century, housewives had extensive knowledge of herbal home remedies. However, much herbal knowledge has been lost because it was not passed down from generation to generation, as it was in traditional cultures. As the twentieth century medical advances became more and more dramatic, the populace assumed a "doctor knows best" attitude, giving up responsibility for and control of their health care. Fortunately, this is now changing. Today, Americans are rediscovering herbal healing with unprecedented enthusiasm. Recent studies show that more than 75 percent of Americans now use some form of alternative healing for their health care, with the result that herbal remedies have become immensely popular as natural health promoters, and as complements to over-the-counter drugstore medicines as well as prescription drugs. Even the American academic establishment is getting into the herbal medicine act, with major U.S.

research centers now investigating the healing potential of herbs and other alternative medical approaches.

An established theory is that herbs can ward off cancer by their indirect stimulation of the immune system, but in recent years, researchers have begun identifying plant components that are actively anticancer. Herbs contain scores of these biologically active chemicals, which may one day prove to have therapeutic uses. Several anticancer drugs have already been derived from plants, the most notable of which is Taxol, from the Pacific yew tree.

The metabolism of nature's intelligence takes place on the level of the neuroreceptors in the human body, which serve as a link between the physical body and the environment in which it lives. The human body possesses a multitude of neuroreceptors that are responsive to biological substances found in herbs. These substances have the capacity of targeting specific receptors within the body. Thus, the health and balance of the body—the *yin* and *yang,* in Chinese terms—is restored through the plant's influence.

Testing the Medical Use of Herbs

It's difficult to scientifically test and evaluate the medical use of herbs in the laboratory. These plants are complex, which may be why they have such a dramatic effect on human physiology. All living things, including humans, are composed of families of related organic compounds. Therefore the proteins, enzymes, sugars, vitamins, minerals, and even toxic substances found in plants can, and will, affect the human system by relating to similar substances found in the body.

FACTS

Colds and flu are generally considered to be due to viral or bacterial infections and are often associated with stress, fatigue, depression, and excess cold or heat.

Frequently, a plant chemical, when applied to the human system, will mimic its own usual reaction inside the plant from which it originated.

A classic example of this reaction is that of antibiotics, which evolved in plants to ward off attacks by specific bacteria and fungi. These substances act the same way in animals. Therefore, it appears that there may be similarly transferable processes between plants and humans.

There are also many subtle similarities between plant and animal biochemistry, beyond the more direct relationship already described. For example, human sex hormones have been discovered in yeast and certain fungi. Several plants contain compounds in themselves that resemble those found naturally in humans, such as the endorphins that inhibit pain.

The World Health Organization (WHO) is making efforts all over the globe to safeguard the kind of medicine, called "folk," or "traditional," on which the bulk of the world's population depends, just as it has for eons. Their continuing fieldwork among indigenous peoples is of great value and is urgently needed. Plant species are disappearing at an alarming rate and can never be replaced. A vast amount of herbal knowledge gained over the centuries is being lost with the disappearance of the forest habitats—especially the rain forests—and the displacement of their inhabitants, whose information about the properties of native and local herbs and plants is often stored in memory, not in written records.

Medicine of the People

Herbalism has always been considered the "medicine of the people." It consists of simple remedies (in medieval times herbs were called "simples") to be used at home to treat minor ailments or wounds. Herbs have also been used as a supplement to prescription drugs given for chronic and acute conditions. Many herbs can be easily prepared as teas, and more complex preparations can be made at home. Most people choose commercially prepared herbal products available at health food stores and some pharmacies. It is important to keep in mind that although most herbs are considered to be safe, they can be potent and should be treated respectfully. Never exceed the recommended dose, and do not continue with home treatment if a condition worsens or becomes chronic. If the true diagnosis is in any way uncertain, a professional should be consulted.

Although some herbs work quickly, especially for acute conditions, chronic problems may require several weeks, or even months, of treatment before significant results are achieved. With herbal treatments, symptoms may change as time progresses, so it is necessary to review the remedy and its effects periodically at least once a month and to be prepared to alter it in accord with changing conditions. Professional herbalists who monitor their patients often adjust their remedies frequently as the person's general state changes. Self-reliance and self-treatment are admirable, but due caution must always be taken, especially if the person is taking any prescription medicines for a particular condition. Some herbs interact with prescription drugs; therefore, you should *always* consult your doctor or health care professional before using herbal remedies in conjunction with prescription medicines.

Playing It Safe

Because herbal medicines have been serving people's health and healing needs for thousands upon thousands of years, we tend to think of them as innocuous and safe. And, by and large, herbal remedies are one of the safest ways to treat most bodily dysfunctions, from the everyday minor ones, such as cuts and scrapes, colds and influenza, menstrual difficulties, and childhood ailments, to more serious conditions, such as chronic arthritis and respiratory problems. Nonetheless, it must be stressed that herbs are not merely helpful plants; they can be potent medicines and, as such, are to be treated with the respect a powerful drug or agent deserves.

Today, we tend to think of herbs as "natural" forms of drugs, but they are actually foods that possess medicinal qualities, and they are ingested into the system (or used topically and absorbed through the skin) just as our ordinary foods are. In fact, many common foods that we don't consider to be "herbal" or healing are now being discovered to possess a wide range of beneficial properties. For example, the common blueberry—the stuff of many homemade cobbler and millions of muffins—has been found to be the most potent antioxidant extant. It outdistances by far the former favorite antioxidant substances that have been highly touted. And the substance lycopene, which is thought to reduce the risk of prostate cancer and inhibit the spread of several types of cancer, including breast cancer, lung cancer, endometrial cancer, and stomach cancer, is found in astonishing abundance in one of our most common vegetables—the tomato! Whoever thought spaghetti drenched in tomato sauce would be good for you? Used as foods or flavoring agents (e.g., garlic, parsley, turmeric), herbs combine with our bodies and are able to address both the symptoms and underlying causes of health problems. Herbs offer the body nutrients it does not always receive but definitely needs. Unfortunately, commercially grown food is often grown on depleted soil as well as doused with pesticides. As we've already mentioned, many people do not pay sufficient attention to proper nutrition because they are "too busy" or simply lack the knowledge or interest. So try to keep herbs in mind as you incorporate proper nutrition into your anti-aging regimen.

Precautions You Can Take

When considering safety, it is important to remember that herbs, when used as medicines, are essentially body balancers that help the body's entire ecosystem to heal itself. If you are going to use herbs medicinally, there are three primary rules you should follow:

1. *Do not self-diagnose.* Even minor conditions could be symptoms of a serious problem. If possible, consult someone who is a natural health care specialist.
2. *Work closely with your health care provider.* If you are under the care of a physician who is giving you prescription drugs, discuss any herbal treatments you are considering with him or her.
3. *Educate yourself about herbs and their uses.* Bookstore shelves are crammed with dozens of books on herbs for every purpose; some are regularly updated with new information.

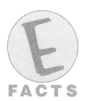

Varicose veins are often a problem for women. Studies have shown that butcher's broom extract can constrict blood vessels. It contains steroid-like compounds that experts believe can inhibit inflammation and shrink swollen varicose veins.

Beware of Possible Side Effects

Generally speaking, herbs provide a rich variety of healing agents and—as most of them are edible plants—they are as safe as foods and have almost no side effects. Of course, one must always consider the individual who is taking the herbs, and for what reasons. Just as some people are allergic to certain foods and have adverse reactions to eating, say, strawberries or eggplant, you must take your own constitution into consideration. If, for example, aspirin upsets your stomach, you would not want to take willow bark, from which aspirin is derived.

The key to avoiding an adverse reaction is in moderation, both in formulation and in dosage. Always follow the dosage recommendations on the labels of any herbal products that you buy and, if you make your own preparations, be sure you have proper directions. Anything mishandled or taken to excess can cause negative side effects, but these are easy enough to avoid with proper attention and care (just as you wash your cutting board after cutting up a raw chicken to avoid contaminating your other foods with bacteria). The use of common sense is as important regarding taking herbs as it is in preparing food, driving your car, working around the house, or any other area of life. Safety is never a guarantee without proper precaution.

However, as a general rule, herbs can be used freely and safely as part of your health regimen, just as you might take a daily multiple vitamin tablet, considering it not as a medicine but as a health benefit for maintenance.

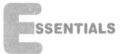 **ESSENTIALS**

According to Daniel Reid in *A Handbook of Healing Chinese Herbs*, "Schisandra has long been popular in Chinese households as an all-round sexual tonic and balanced energy rejuvenation for both men and women. It lends itself well to use in tonic longevity formulas. This herb is widely used for its balanced energies and broad spectrum of therapeutic effects."

Herbs for Common Ailments

The whole idea of herbal remedies really isn't as "new agey" as you may believe. In fact, herbs can be used to treat any number of ailments, including several common conditions of aging. From something as simple as the common cold, to something as complex as varicose veins, there are several well-known herbal remedies to help you out.

Allergies	Alfalfa, Burdock, Comfrey, Echinacea, Goldenseal, and Ma Huang (Ephedra)
Anorexia nervosa	Chamomile, Dandelion, Kelp, Lady's Slipper, Licorice, Passionflower, Skullcap, Red Clover, Wild Yam, and Yellow Dock
Arthritis	Alfalfa, Devil's Claw, Echinacea, White Willow, and Yucca
Asthma	Alfalfa, Asthma Weed, Capsicum, Chlorophyll, Cascara Sagrada, Comfrey, Fenugreek, Garlic, Hops, Licorice, Ma Huang (Ephedra), and Slippery Elm
Back pain	Alfalfa, Comfrey, Horsetail, Oatstraw, and Slippery Elm
Baldness	Aloe Vera, Horsetail, Jojoba, Kelp, and Oatstraw
Body odor	Chlorophyll
Bronchitis	Elecampane, Nettle, White Horehound, Cowslip, and Thyme
Bruises	Black Walnut, Comfrey, Dandelion, Horsetail, Kelp, Rose Hips, Slippery Elm, White Oak, and Yellow Dock
Burns	Aloe Vera, Comfrey, Horsetail, and Slippery Elm

Cancer	Alfalfa, Astragalus, Burdock Root, Chaparral, Echinacea, Garlic, Onion, Ginkgo Biloba, Ginseng, Goldenseal, and Turmeric
Cholesterol reduction	Angelica, Black Cohosh, Hawthorn, Hawthorn and Walnut (combination), and Mistletoe
Cold sores	Aloe Vera, Capsicum (Cayenne), Comfrey, Garlic, Goldenseal, White Oak Bark, and Myrrh (in topical alcohol solution)
Common cold	Alfalfa or Peppermint (teas), Raspberry (tea), Aloe Vera (drink), Echinacea, Fenugreek, Garlic, Ginger (settles stomach), Goldenseal, Kelp, Rose Hips, and Slippery Elm (for coughs and sore throat)
Constipation	Cascara Sagrada, Comfrey, Garlic, Psyllium, Slippery Elm, and Triphala
Diabetes	Alfalfa, Burdock, Garlic, Goldenseal, Red Clover, Uva Ursi, Watercress, and Yellow Dock
Diarrhea	Alfalfa, Glucomannan, Raspberry (tea), and Slippery Elm
Dieting and obesity	Bladderwrack (Fucus), Kelp, Garlic, Glucomannan, and Ma Huang (Ephedra)
Digestive disorders	Angelica, Anise, Chamomile, Comfrey, Calamus Root (tea), Dandelion, Fennel, Garlic, Ginger Root, Goldenseal, Papaya or Aloe Vera (with meals), Peppermint, and Slippery Elm
Dry skin	Alfalfa and Aloe Vera
Energy	Fo-Ti, Ginseng, Gotu Kola

Fatigue	Capsicum (Cayenne), Ginseng, American Ginseng and Red Deer Antler (combination), Gotu Kola, and Oats
Flatulence	Alfalfa, Anise, Blessed Thistle, Capsicum (Cayenne), Caraway, Fennel, Garlic, Goldenseal, Peppermint, and Wild Yam
Flu	Garlic and Symfre
Gallstones	Chamomile, Dandelion, and Yellow Dock
Gout	Burdock Root, Colchicum (tincture), Guggula, Celery, and White Bryony (tincture—for pain)
Gray hair	Mulberry Fruit, Privet, Eclipta, Yin Tonics (in general)
Gum disease	Capsicum (Cayenne), Coneflower, Goldenseal, and Myrrh
Headache	Chamomile, Feverfew, Hops, Peppermint plus Catnip (tea for headaches of stomach origin), Red Sage, Skullcap, Spearmint (tea), White Willow, and Wood Betony
Heartburn	Aloe Vera, Burnet, Gentian, and Peppermint
Hemorrhoids	Stone Root (capsule and suppository) and Goldenseal (suppository)
Hives	Alfalfa, Caltrop, Chamomile, Echinacea, Ginseng, Licorice, Sarsaparilla, and Yellow Dock
Hypertension	Cayenne (Capsicum), Garlic, Glucomannan, Hawthorn Berries, Hibiscus Flowers, Hops, Lady's Slipper, Passionflower, Skullcap, and Valerian

Immune deficiency	Alfalfa, Chaparral, Echinacea, Garlic, and Pau D'Arco
Indigestion	Anise, Fennel, Peppermint, and Spearmint
Insect bites	Aloe Vera (gel), Comfrey, Feverfew, and Papaya (for insect bites); Tea Tree Oil and Goldenseal (as insect repellents)
Insomnia	Catnip, Chamomile, Hops, Lady's Slipper, Skullcap, and Valerian Root
Memory	Astragalus, Calamus, Cayenne, Dong Quai, Ginkgo Biloba Leaf Extract, Ginger, Ginseng, Gotu Kola, and Red Deer Antler
Mental health	Cayenne, Ginseng, Gotu Kola
Nasal congestion	Comfrey, Coneflower (*Echinacea angustifolium*), Eucalyptus, Fenugreek, and Magnolia Blossoms (tea)
Night blindness	Bilberry
Osteoporosis	Comfrey and Horsetail
Pain	Black Cohosh Root, Bugleweed, Catnip, Chaparral, Comfrey, Cornsilk, Fenugreek, Hops, Lady's Slipper, Mullein, Paul D'Arco, Valerian, White Willow Bark, Wild Yam (muscle pain), and Wintergreen
Prostate trouble	Capsicum (Cayenne), False Unicorn Root, Goldenseal, Juniper Berries, Saw Palmetto Berries (oil extract), Siberian Ginseng, and Uva Ursi
Psoriasis	Burdock Root, Chickweed, Common Figwort, Mullein, Slippery Elm (tea), and Yellow American Saffron (tea)

Skin problems	Alfalfa, Aloe Vera, Burdock, Comfrey, Dandelion, Goldenseal, Horsetail, Oatstraw, Queen of the Meadow, Yarrow, and Yellow Dock
Smoking	Hops, Skullcap, Valerian, Catnip, and Slippery Elm
Stress	Alfalfa, Chamomile, Ginseng, Gotu Kola, Hops, Kelp, Lady's Slipper, Passionflower, and Valerian
Tonsillitis and sore throat	Echinacea, Bayberry Root, Ginger Root, Goldenseal (gargle), Marigold Flowers (tincture as throat swab), Pleurisy Root, and St. John's Wort
Tooth decay	Horsetail and Peppermint Oil (toothache)
Urinary tract infections	Barberry (Uva Ursi) (tincture), Buchu, Couch Grass (tincture), Echinacea, Garlic, Goldenseal (tea), Juniper Berries, Parsley Root and Seed (tea or tincture)
Varicose veins	Butcher's Broom, Capsicum (Cayenne), Goldenseal, Horsetail, Kelp, Oatstraw, Parsley, White Oak Bark, and Witch Hazel

ESSENTIALS

If you want to gather your own herbs, you must be able to identify the plants properly. To do this, you will need a field guide. The best is *A Field Guide to Medicinal Plants: Eastern and Central North America,* by noted herbalists Steven Foster and James A. Duke, Ph.D. This book discusses more than 500 pen-and-ink drawings and 200 color plates.

Herbal Remedies for Osteoarthritis and Rheumatism

There are two main types of arthritis: osteoarthritis (OA), which is characterized by pain and swelling of the joints, generally due to wear and tear, and rheumatoid arthritis (RA), which is characterized by the inflammation of many joints and requires professional treatment. Rheumatism is a general term for any muscle pain; lumbago is lower-back pain. Symptoms often worsen in damp weather. These are the key symptoms:

- Stiffness and joint pain
- Swollen or deformed joints
- Hot or burning sensations in joints (RA)
- Creaking sounds in joints

And here are some herbal remedies to help you out:

- *Angelica* is a warming and stimulating herb effective for "cold" types of osteoarthritis and for rheumatism.
- *Devil's claw* has a potent and anti-inflammatory action that has been compared to cortisone. It's better for osteoarthritis and degenerative conditions than for rheumatoid arthritis.
- *Bogbean* is a cleansing, cooling, and anti-inflammatory herb useful for "hotter" types of arthritis and for muscle pain.
- *White willow* is rich in salicylates, which are anti-inflammatories that cool hot joints; it's especially useful for the pain associated with the acute phases of arthritis and for muscle pain

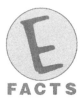

FACTS

Herbs are used to provide the body with the ideal environment to promote health and self-healing. Some herbs may be taken on a daily basis for overall good health; others are added in times of poor health to strengthen a body system.

Amazing Garlic

Garlic, one of the world's most popular culinary herbs, also has a long history as a medicinal plant. Indeed, scientific studies have verified what herbalists have known for centuries—that garlic both prevents and treats illness in a wide variety of ways.

Among its many attributes, garlic is known to lower cholesterol levels, thin the blood, kill bacteria, boost the immune system, lower blood sugar levels, and reduce risk of certain types of cancer. There is also evidence that the herb helps relieve asthma, ease ear infections, and facilitate healthy cell function. Bottom line: Garlic should be consumed often by those who want to maintain their health and age well.

How to Obtain Healing Herbs

There are three ways to obtain healing herbs: gather them in the wild, grow them yourself, or buy them. Since most people will choose to buy ready-made preparations in their health food stores or from mail-order sources rather than either gathering or growing them, there are some pointers to use when buying medicinal herbs:

- Whenever possible, buy fresh herbs that are organically grown or wild crafted (grown in their natural habitat). When buying fresh-dried herbs, make sure they are grown locally.
- If buying bulk herbs, test a sample by rubbing some between your fingers to check the smell. Even dried herbs when crushed give off strong evidence of their volatile oils, and so potency is easily evident.
- Buy the best quality herbs available. Bargain herbs are usually adulterated. More costly products from reputable companies are a better choice because the growing/gathering/preparation/storage phases of the process are supported by experience and quality control.
- When choosing packaged herbs, buy from a company that specializes in herbs, not one that is primarily a supplier of vitamins or other supplements. Herbal companies tend to be devotees of their products and have a high level of integrity in handling and preparation.

- Make sure that any product you buy is tightly sealed and has been kept away from excess light and heat. Check the expiration date.
- Ask your herbal consultant or health care practitioner what brands he or she recommends.
- Do not rely on information about herbs from a clerk in a health food store or pharmacy, especially if it is part of a large chain store. Ask to see the buyer of herbal products or the store manager if you want information. You can also ask whether they have a qualified herbalist on staff or can recommend someone who practices herbalism locally. Such a person would likely be a regular customer.

CHAPTER 5
Anti-aging Tactics

There's more to anti-aging than just watching what you eat and exercising enough. Though these are certainly important, not only for your anti-aging regimen, but also for your health, there are a few other tactics that will help you to feel young. This chapter is going to help you to recognize the importance of breaking bad habits and setting up good habits, as well as address the issues of stress, sex, and depression as they relate to aging.

It's Never Too Late to Think Young

Is it possible to slow or even reverse the aging process once we're fully in its grip? You bet! Contrary to popular belief, it's never too late to "think young" by breaking bad lifestyle habits and improving our environmental conditions. Everything we do that's good for our bodies and minds helps reverse the bad.

Take smoking, for example. Many long-time smokers refuse to quit under the erroneous assumption that the damage is already done. However, numerous clinical studies have shown that our bodies begin repairing the damage to our respiratory system within days of that last cigarette. Unless you already have cancer or emphysema, the health of your lungs (and other organs adversely affected by tobacco, such as the heart) will continue to improve until, finally, you're almost as well as before you took that first puff.

And let's not forget the gradual reversal of the cosmetic effects—stained teeth and fingers, facial wrinkles, bad breath, and the constant stench of smoke on your person—of smoking. There's no question that by merely kicking the tobacco habit, you're giving your body a new lease on life.

Diet is another aspect of the aging equation that's never too late to change. As we've already discussed, the harmful effects of a poor diet—that is, too much red meat and fried, fatty foods and too few fruits and vegetables—are almost too numerous to count. A lousy diet (which often results from having too little time to cook properly) can be a springboard for a wide variety of age-related problems, including atherosclerosis, hypertension, heart disease, diabetes, osteoporosis, a weakened immune response, and even cancer.

But as with smoking, a simple change in dietary habits can have a remarkable effect on your health and, in turn, how you age—no matter how old you are when you start. For most people, a change for the better can be seen simply by eating less red meat and fatty foods and more fresh vegetables and fruits. This reduces the amount of cholesterol in your system, gives your body the vitamins and minerals it needs to function well, and packs your system with antioxidants and other anti-aging compounds.

Finally, let's consider the issue of exercise. We all know that regular exercise is good for us, but few of us actually take the time to fit physical activity into our busy schedules. Older people, in particular, are often reluctant to exercise, for fear of injuring themselves, yet they need it just as much, if not more, than men and women who are younger. In the older population, exercise keeps the heart and lungs working at full capacity, the muscles well toned, the bones strong, and the immune system in tip-top shape. Exercise also helps maintain mental clarity and, when done in a group setting, allows you to remain socially active.

FACTS

The proportion of older people is considerably higher among whites than in minority populations. This reflects an overall trend that has changed very little throughout American history. For each group, the approximate percentages of men and women sixty-five years or older are:

- Caucasian—13 percent
- African-American—8 percent
- Hispanic—5 percent
- Other—7 percent

The problem, though, is that in the minds of many seniors, exercise is defined as weight lifting, running, tennis, cycling—activities that may be well beyond their ability. But any doctor will tell you that such a definition is incorrect. In truth, anything that keeps you active and gets the heart rate up counts as exercise. Walk around the block a couple of times, exercise in a pool, go dancing, play golf. Your goal isn't to look like Arnold Schwarzenegger but to keep your body active, strong, and young. And it's easier than you might think.

Is it ever too late to think young? Absolutely not. All you need is the right attitude and a strong desire to stay healthy and vibrant. The moral is simple: Think young, act young, stay young.

Getting a Good Night's Sleep

Do you get a good night's sleep? Do you awaken every morning feeling rested and refreshed? If you're like most people, your answer is probably no.

Insomnia is one of the most prevalent problems in the United States, and one of the most common reasons people see a doctor. It's estimated that one in four American adults and one in two seniors experience occasional or recurrent sleep problems, and those figures will continue to rise as the baby boomer generation reaches old age.

Sleep disturbances—more commonly known under the umbrella term "insomnia"—can be caused by a host of reasons, including depression and chronic pain, but a hectic lifestyle is probably the most common. This is especially true among families that have infants or small children. There never seems to be enough hours in the day to get everything done, so our daily schedule intrudes into our nighttime schedule. When we finally do get to bed, our minds race, and it's 2 A.M. before we finally doze off into a fitful sleep.

Sleep disturbances are more than a minor inconvenience; severe, chronic insomnia can have a devastating effect on physical and mental well-being, which in turn can have a dramatic influence on aging. Even occasional insomnia can affect our health to some degree, including a weakening of the immune system.

Most people assume they need a minimum of eight hours of sleep to feel good, but in truth everyone has different sleep requirements. Most healthy adults sleep an average of seven to eight hours a night, though some people do well with a little more or a little less slumber.

Following are some helpful tips on how to maintain healthy sleep patterns:

- *Reduce the amount of stress and anxiety in your life.* Stress is one of the most common causes of transient insomnia; it keeps the brain awake and functioning long into the night or wee hours of the morning. Stress causes worry, and worry interferes with sleep. Acknowledging the problem is the first step, followed by a resolution to take care of those problems you can and a promise not to dwell on those you can't. (We'll discuss stress in more detail later in this chapter.)

- *Maintain a healthy lifestyle.* This means eating right and exercising regularly. But sleep specialists warn that you should not exercise immediately before bedtime. Physical activity tends to stimulate the body rather than relax it. Exercise in the morning or after work, but save the evening for relaxation.

- *Establish a sleep schedule.* Determine the best time for you to go to sleep (it's different for everyone and depends on how much sleep you need to feel rested and alert the next day) and try to go to bed at exactly that time every evening. A soothing bedtime ritual can also help.

- *Use your bed only for sleep.* Watching TV, reading, and eating are best done in the living room—not the bedroom. The goal is to quickly prepare your body for sleep when you finally go to bed. If you find that you haven't fallen asleep within twenty minutes, get up and do something else, such as reading or balancing your checkbook.

- *Make sure your bed is comfortable.* A bed that is too hard or too soft can have a serious effect on your ability to fall asleep and stay asleep. When shopping for a new mattress, check out as many different kinds as you can before making your decision. Never buy the first mattress you see, and never buy a mattress without lying on it for several minutes to determine how it feels. Your pillow should be equally comfortable, neither too soft nor too hard.

- *Make sure your bedroom is conducive to sleep.* Many people sleep poorly because their bedroom is too noisy, too bright, too hot, or too cold. Some people can sleep under almost any conditions, but most of us need darkness and comfort for a truly restful night's sleep. Soundproof your bedroom if you're bothered by outside noise and use blackout curtains to keep out intrusive light. And don't forget the small things; the light from a seemingly harmless clock face can inhibit sleep in sensitive individuals.

- *Don't linger in bed after the alarm goes off.* Hitting the snooze button every morning can wreak havoc with your internal clock and make you feel tired and listless all day long. Establishing a set time to get up each morning keeps your body clock in sync and ensures restful sleep.

- *Avoid alcohol and tobacco.* Alcohol may make you drowsy, but it interferes with brain activity and actually impairs sleep. Nicotine is a powerful stimulant; it's the last thing you need if you suffer from insomnia.
- *Skip late-night snacks.* A stomach full of food can interfere with sleep by forcing the body to work when it should be resting. In addition, greasy foods can cause indigestion.
- *Consider an herbal supplement to help you sleep.* Both valerian and kava kava have been shown to induce sleep among people with occasional insomnia. Melatonin can also be effective.

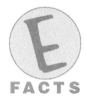

FACTS

More than 23 million Americans experience some form of anxiety, making it one of the most common psychological illnesses in the nation.

The Effects of Stress on Health and Aging

Stress is an unavoidable part of life. Whether you live in the city or the country, are rich or poor, male or female, black or white, there's no escaping it. The best we can do is try to minimize the stress in our lives and take steps to keep it from affecting our health. Bottom line: Chronic, unrelenting stress damages our health and causes us to age much faster.

Though you may not realize it, there are actually two kinds of stress in our lives—good stress and bad stress. Good stress is the excitement/anxiety we feel when our favorite sports team tries to rally during the closing minutes of the game. Our heart races, our palms get sweaty, our breathing becomes a little labored. However, this physical response seldom lasts very long and thus does us little harm (aside, perhaps, from a sore throat from shouting our team to a last-minute victory).

Bad stress results in the same physical reaction but comes from physical or mental discomfort, such as that caused by a near accident on the highway, rumors that your company is about to go belly-up, or a serious illness. Unlike the sources of good stress, bad stress can become long term, hitting us day after day without a break, until we become physically ill and mentally drained.

Simply speaking, stress readies the body's fight-or-flight mechanism, a primitive reaction that aided in our prehistoric ancestors' day-to-day survival. However, modern stress is seldom resolved by either of those reactions; we can't fight it, and we can't run from it. It's just there, every day, perniciously affecting our health and well-being.

Stress results in a number of intriguing physical responses. As the fight-or-flight mechanism is triggered, hormone production kicks into overdrive, filling our bloodstreams with a wide variety of chemicals. Our blood pressure skyrockets, proteins are turned into sugars for fast fuel, and, depending on the circumstances, we may even experience a brief period of amazing strength, which explains those tales of women lifting cars at the scene of an accident.

If, by some chance, our lives are relatively stress free, then the occasional stressful event will have little lasting impact on our health. Once the stressful issue is resolved, our bodies return to normal and everything is fine. However, for most Americans, stress is an everyday occurrence, and that's not good. Repeated stress can stimulate the production of cell-damaging free radicals, depress the immune system, increase blood pressure, raise blood cholesterol levels, boost anxiety levels, and promote depression. Common health problems caused or made worse by stress include the following:

- Headaches
- Neck and back problems
- Heart irregularities
- Skin disorders such as hives and rashes
- Digestive problems
- Menstrual difficulties
- Insomnia
- Fatigue
- More frequent colds and sore throats
- Mood swings

Furthermore, a growing body of clinical data suggests that chronic stress robs the body of vitamins, minerals, and other nutrients. As a result, many doctors now prescribe nutritional supplements for their patients who are under aggravated stress due to their work, illness, or other problems. Antioxidants such as beta carotene and vitamins C and E may also be needed to combat the increased production of free radicals caused by chronic stress.

FACTS

According to the U.S. Department of Health, Education and Welfare, an estimated 23 percent of all persons aged sixty-five to seventy-four years have a hearing impairment, and 40 percent of those seventy-five and older have a hearing loss.

Stress also affects our behavior and lifestyle, almost always negatively. When under stress, we tend to look for easy solutions, such as alcohol or recreational drugs. People who smoke tend to do so more often when under stress, and it's not uncommon for women to develop eating disorders such as anorexia or bulimia. The trouble is that once we start these behaviors, it's difficult to stop when our stress levels go down.

Stress Reduction Made Easy

If you're like most Americans, stress is an everyday part of your life. And chances are, it's affecting your health to some degree and, thus, how well you'll age and how long you'll live. While it's impossible to completely eliminate stress from our lives, there are ways to reduce its effects on our minds and bodies. Following are some helpful stress-reduction tips:

- *Get a checkup.* If you've been under a lot of stress for a long time, it's important that you find out how it has affected your health and what you need to do to reduce its impact. Your doctor can pinpoint specific stress-related problems and offer advice on how to correct them.
- *Don't hold in stress-related issues.* Talking with family and close friends about the stressful issues in your life can go a long way

toward making them more manageable. If necessary, consider seeking professional counseling.

- *Spend quality time with your closest friends.*
- *Fix it or forget it.* Do what you can to resolve the stressful situations in your life and stop worrying about those you can't resolve. After all, what's the sense of losing sleep and harming your health dwelling on things over which you have no control?
- *Get plenty of exercise.* Physical activity stimulates the production of hormones that relieve stress, diminish anxiety, and improve mood.
- *Pursue a hobby.* A calming activity such as gardening or painting is a great way to forget your troubles.
- *Get a pet.* Playing with a cat, dog, or hamster can be very calming.
- *Get away for a while.* Sometimes our environment is the biggest stressor in our lives. If it's been a while since you've taken a vacation, get as far away from the source of your troubles as you can and enjoy yourself. Most importantly, don't take your problems with you! Leave work at the office and home problems at the front door.
- *Take good care of your finances and do what you can to minimize debt.* Financial problems are one of the leading causes of stress, not to mention marital problems.
- *Don't assume other people's problems.* Charity is good, but you should think first of yourself and your family.
- *Take up meditation and other stress-reducing techniques.* Fifteen minutes of uninterrupted meditation is a wonderful way to melt away the day's worries and stress.
- *Try aromatherapy.* Many essential oils, such as lavender, have proven stress-reducing qualities. A warm, lavender-scented bath, for example, is a great way to relax and unwind. It also promotes restful sleep.
- *Improve your time management at work and at home so that you're not constantly playing catch-up.* Reducing "office rush" is an important way of reducing stress.
- *Laugh!* It really is the best medicine—for both our minds and our bodies.
- *Avoid harmful solutions, such as drinking alcohol and taking drugs.* Alcohol is a depressant that will make the problems in your life worse and, thus, increase your stress levels.

- *Reduce your caffeine intake.* Caffeine is a stimulant that agitates the body and exacerbates the perception of the stress in our lives.
- *Learn to assert yourself when necessary.* People will walk all over you if allowed to, and that can add a lot of stress to your life.

Relaxation: What It Can Do for You

Some people are naturally hyper; others are made that way by the stress in their lives. The inability to relax at the end of the day can maintain dangerously high levels of stress, which in turn can adversely affect our health. Following are some tried-and-true relaxation techniques guaranteed to help you relax and feel better.

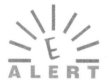

Don't forget your immunizations!

- *Influenza vaccine.* Often considered a minor inconvenience, influenza results in 20,000 deaths each year.
- *Pneumonia vaccine.* More than 70,000 American deaths are attributed to pneumococcal infections each year, so a regular pneumonia shot is a good idea for everyone over sixty-five years old and those who are in high-risk groups.
- *Hepatitis B vaccine.* As many as 300,000 Americans are infected with hepatitis B each year, and more than a million people are chronic carriers.
- *Measles/mumps/rubella.* Most children receive this series of vaccinations prior to entering school, but if you were born after 1956 and are unsure of whether you were vaccinated, it might be a good idea to get one.

The Power of a Massage

Few things are more soothing than being rubbed the right way! A regular massage can ease stress, relax tense muscles, and help your worries melt away. And you don't have to spend a lot of money on a professional masseuse to reap these benefits; a deep back and shoulder rub from your spouse can have the same remarkable benefits.

For best results, make sure your environment is relaxing. Dim the lights, put on some soft music, and light some fragrant candles (lavender, chamomile, and sandalwood are all good choices). Lightly warm some massage oil (or even baby oil or a light vegetable oil, if you don't have any commercial massage oil) and have your partner massage your neck, shoulders, back, and legs with strong, deep motions. Working out the kinks may hit some sensitive pressure points, but a massage should not be overly painful.

Many people consider massage an indulgence, but it actually offers a lot of medical benefits. A growing number of hospitals routinely massage patients suffering from a wide variety of ailments, and studies have found that massage can improve the cognitive function of nursing home patients, as well as maintain the elasticity of aging skin. In addition, massage has been found effective in helping certain premature babies grow and thrive. So don't look at massage as an occasional gift; look at it as a necessary part of staying healthy and youthful.

Easing Your Mind

The concept of meditation as a relaxation technique still feels uncomfortably "new agey" to a lot of people. But in truth, it's centuries old—and very effective, especially for people who encounter stress daily as part of their jobs.

Consider meditation a simple form of self-hypnosis. By sitting comfortably in a calm environment and focusing on a single relaxing word—called a mantra—you are, in a sense, "forcing" yourself to relax and calm down. It's relatively easy to learn and a terrific way to stay focused and calm even during periods of extreme stress.

For best results, try to find a twenty-minute period in which you can be alone. Some people like to meditate before they go to work; others find it more effective to meditate when they get home or later in the evening. Everyone is different, and you'll have to determine which time works best for you. Make sure your environment is quiet—no phones or TV—and that you won't be interrupted during this special time.

FACTS

Researchers at the Medical College of Georgia report that transcendental meditation can help lower blood pressure by reducing constriction of the blood vessels. Longtime practitioners, they found, were able to relax their blood vessels by a much as 6.5 percent during meditation.

Sit comfortably with your legs crossed, close your eyes, and concentrate on your mantra. Simple, calming words or phrases work best, such as *quiet field* or *stillness*. Repeat your mantra over and over, blocking out everything else that wants to intrude. If your mind starts to wander, refocus on your mantra. As you do this, your mind and body will enter a comforting state of calm, and you'll feel the stress and anxiety in your life melt away. By doing this daily, the negative impacts of stress on your health and well-being can be substantially decreased.

How does meditation help the mind and body? Studies have found that effective meditation actually slows your heart rate, lowers blood pressure, increases blood flow to the brain, and balances brain wave patterns. It also boosts the immune system and improves cognitive function, including memory.

Once you become adept at meditating, don't hesitate to take quick five-minute "calming breaks" throughout a stressful day. If you work in an office, simply close your door, tell your secretary you don't want to be bothered for five minutes, shut your eyes, and focus on your mantra. Within just a few minutes you should feel rested, relaxed, and ready to get on with business.

Making Your Senses Work for You

Most people take for granted the many scents and fragrances we encounter throughout the day, never realizing that odors can help us relax, improve our mood, and even help us sleep. This concept is known as aromatherapy, and it's rapidly becoming one of the fastest-growing fields in natural medicine. Why? Because it really works. And it costs just pennies.

It's common knowledge that certain fragrances can quickly lift us from a foul mood. If you don't believe this is so, consider the smile that crosses your face when you inhale the yummy scent of a freshly baked pie, or your partner's perfume or cologne. Other mood boosters include the scent of pine (which is a holiday favorite), cinnamon, mint, and pumpkin.

There are a large number of relaxing aromatic oils on the market, but the best include lavender, sage, sandalwood, frankincense, and chamomile. How you use them is up to you. Some people light scented candles as they relax after a hard day's work or place fragrant potpourri throughout their home. Others prefer to place a few drops of scented oils in their water while they relax in a hot bath or a few drops of scented oil on their pillow to help them unwind and fall asleep faster at night.

The important thing is to select a fragrance that is both appealing and relaxing. Floral scents tend to work best, because food scents can make us hungry. Avoid tart or biting fragrances, such as lemon, because they may have the opposite effect, perking you up instead of calming you down. You may have to experiment until you find the scent that is right for you, but it's well worth the effort.

Beating the Blues

Depression is one of the most common mental illnesses in the world. It afflicts people of all ages and walks of life, and can have a dramatic impact on our overall mental and physical health if not treated.

FACTS

Social support can make a substantial difference between life and death when it comes to recovering from serious illness. Here's proof: A study at Stanford University in Palo Alto, California, found that women with breast cancer who joined a support group lived twice as long as patients who received only medical care.

Almost everyone feels "down in the dumps" once in a while. That's normal and nothing to worry about. But when a feeling of sadness, melancholy, or hopelessness lasts more than two weeks, it becomes a medical issue with far-reaching consequences and should be addressed by a physician. Most cases of clinical depression are the result of a biochemical imbalance in the brain and a psychological imbalance in thinking and can usually be treated with medication, therapy, or a combination of both.

The most important thing you must understand is that depression is not a personal failing. It is not caused by something you did or did not do, nor is it something you could have prevented. Depression happens, and it happens a lot. By recognizing the most common symptoms, you can determine early on whether you or a loved one has clinical depression and then seek help. Symptoms include the following:

- A change in eating or sleeping habits
- Inability to concentrate or difficulty in making decisions
- Withdrawal from friends, family, or other social contacts
- Preoccupation with aches and pains; persistent headaches or stomachaches, or chronic pain
- Persistent sadness or hopelessness; frequent crying for no apparent reason
- General irritability or restlessness
- Decreased energy or fatigue
- Feelings of worthlessness, that no one loves you, or that life isn't worth living
- Thoughts of death or suicide, or suicide attempts

If you or someone you care about exhibits three or more of these symptoms, see your doctor immediately for a full evaluation. Depression reacts very well to a large number of medications, and symptoms usually subside relatively quickly once treatment begins.

Sex and Longevity

Sex not only feels good, it's good for you. Regular sexual activity benefits the mind and body in a variety of ways and ultimately can help you live longer.

This isn't just theory; it's clinical fact. A Duke University longitudinal study on aging found a strong correlation between the frequency and enjoyment of sexual intercourse and longevity. And a more recent British study had the same result, noting lower overall rates of mortality among men who have sex far more frequently than the once-a-week national average.

Bottom line: Men and women who have frequent, loving sex tend to live longer than those who don't.

Working with Your Partner

It's easy to fall into a rut in a long-term relationship, doing the same thing over and over until sex becomes more of a chore than a pleasure. When this happens, both partners may find that their libidos start to ebb, and sex often gets put on the back burner. In extreme cases, weeks and even months may pass between romantic interludes.

This negates all of the healthful effects of regular sexual relations. But keeping the passion in a long-term relationship isn't as difficult as you may think. All it takes is the will and desire.

Sex becomes humdrum for a variety of reasons. The most common include the following:

- *Laziness.* Very often couples develop a technique in the bedroom that initially pleases both partners, and they stick with it to the exclusion of anything else. Once a pattern is established, it takes some work to break it, and many couples find it easier to rely on the tried and true than experiment with something different.
- *Poor communication.* Many couples find it difficult to sit down and discuss their sexual wants and needs, particularly if they were raised in an environment in which sex was a taboo subject. Rather than openly and honestly talking about what they like, they hope and pray that their partner will figure it out for themselves. But this almost never happens. In many cases, a failure to communicate can lead to bedroom frustration and hurt feelings, which only exacerbate the initial problem.
- *Lack of time.* This is one of the most common sexual problems facing couples today. We're simply too busy to enjoy leisurely romance, so we do it on the fly. However, rushed sex can be less satisfying than no sex at all. Sex therapists call this "Social Security Sex"—you get a little bit every month, but it's seldom enough to live on.
- *Children.* As all parents will attest, having a child can put a serious crimp on your sex life. Once you bring the baby home, your time is

so micromanaged that sex can easily become a distant memory. Unfortunately, this can create a pattern that is difficult to break. New parents must learn early that spending some romantic time with each other is just as important as spending time with their newest addition.

As already noted, communication is vital to a strong and satisfying sex life. Couples must learn to be open with each other in discussing what they want, what they don't want, and—most importantly—what they can do to keep their relationship vibrant and exciting. Sex should be spontaneous, but there's nothing wrong with literally scheduling some time together, especially if both partners work long hours. If you have to, make a date on the calendar for dinner and romance—and keep it. Do this as often as you can.

A second honeymoon is another great way to jumpstart a flagging sexual relationship. This means getting away from the house, kids, and work and doing nothing but getting reacquainted in the bedroom. Order room service, play fun bedroom games, take romantic walks, enjoy an expensive meal. The vacation doesn't have to be lengthy—a long weekend will do—but it should involve nothing but love and passion.

Sex and Aging

It's a common misconception that growing older automatically means an end to sexual activity. According to Masters and Johnson and a host of other sex researchers, pleasurable sex can continue well into our seventies, eighties, and beyond. In fact, theoretically we should be able to enjoy sex throughout our entire lives, as long as we are physically healthy. However, one cliché about sex and aging is true—if you don't use it, you'll lose it.

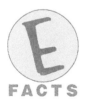

If you want to improve your sex life, give up cigarettes. That's the advice of researchers at the Andrology Institute of America, who found that smokers tend to have sex less frequently than nonsmokers. The researchers also found that habitual smoking damages sperm quality in several ways, from motility to longevity.

Sex holds tremendous value as we grow older. It helps maintain a strong, loving bond with our partner, benefits us physically in a variety of ways, and keeps us feeling young and vital. But while we should never stop enjoying sex, we must recognize the impact the physical changes of age can have on sexual activity. For example, postmenopausal women may experience diminished lubrication and a thinning of the vaginal tissue that can make sexual intercourse uncomfortable (a problem easily solved with the use of a commercial sexual lubricant such as KY Jelly or Astroglide). And men sixty and older may find that their erection is not as hard as it used to be, nor their orgasm as intense. Older men are also more prone to episodes of sexual dysfunction (especially if they smoke or take a lot of different medications), require more time to reach complete arousal, and require more time between sexual encounters.

Physical issues aside, one of the greatest enemies of sexual enjoyment in our later years is inactivity. This is true for both men and women. It's easy to buy into the myth that older people simply don't want or need sex, but in so doing, we deny ourselves one of the greatest pleasures we can ever experience. Following are a few tips for older lovers:

- *Take your time.* Enjoy each other's bodies, make pillow talk, and revel in your intimacy. Sex shouldn't be rushed.
- *Don't agonize over the occasional bout of sexual dysfunction.* It's natural and to be expected, especially as we age. However, if it becomes chronic, consult a urologist to find out why it is happening and what can be done about it. Very often sexual dysfunction can be alleviated simply by switching medications.
- *Be aware of your physical limitations.* Some of the sexual positions you enjoyed at age twenty can be difficult and even painful at age sixty. Experiment to find out what works best for both of you.
- *Practice safe sex.* This is especially true if you are not in a long-term, monogamous relationship. Just because you're older doesn't mean you can't contract a sexually transmitted disease. More than 10 percent of AIDS cases in the United States are people fifty-five and older.
- *Embrace your sexuality; don't hide from it.* Humans are sexual creatures, and sex is a natural part of life. Enjoy this special gift.

Protecting Yourself from the Sun

Most people see the sun as a friend, the giver of warmth, light, and physical and mental well-being. But while the human body needs a certain amount of sunlight to function properly, too much sun exposure can facilitate the aging process as well as increase our risk of skin cancer.

Researchers estimate that as much as 70 percent of skin damage that leads to premature aging comes from excessive sun exposure. For most people, this begins in childhood (approximately 80 percent of sun exposure occurs before age eighteen) and continues well into adulthood, with an increasingly dangerous cumulative effect. Fair-skinned people, those who received repeated sunburns in childhood, and individuals who work out in the sun for several hours every day, such as landscapers, are most at risk.

Many people think a deep suntan is a thing of beauty, but in fact it wreaks havoc with your skin by forcing it to produce more melanin—a natural sun block that the skin produces to keep out damaging ultraviolet rays. Every time you get a sun tan, you're damaging your skin even more. After a while, the skin loses its suppleness, resulting in unsightly wrinkles, leathery skin, and sagging.

Worse, though, is the increased risk of skin cancer—including potentially deadly melanoma. According to the American Cancer Society, the United States sees over 1 million new cases of skin cancer annually, and more than 40,000 of them involve melanoma. Other common skin cancers include basal cell carcinoma and squamous cell carcinoma.

What can you do to decrease your risk? Plenty, say doctors. Foremost, limit your exposure to sunlight. If you must work outdoors, do so in the early morning and late afternoon, when the sun is past its peak. Wear a hat, long pants, and a long-sleeved shirt whenever possible, and cover exposed skin with sunscreen. Sunscreen is especially important when spending time at the beach or at a pool; reapply every time you return from the water.

And don't think you can cheat cancer and still get a great tan by using a tanning booth. Skin damage is skin damage, whether it's achieved by natural or artificial means.

Kicking the Tobacco Habit and Staying Healthy

It is often said that it's more difficult to kick tobacco than heroin. However, that doesn't mean you shouldn't try—and keep trying until you finally succeed. Your health and your very life are at stake.

Do we really need to mention just how bad smoking is for you? A glance at the warnings on all cigarette packages pretty much tells the story. Still, let's take a quick look at why you should quit (and then we'll talk about how):

- Smoking is a major contributor to the five leading causes of death in the United States—heart disease, stroke, cancer (specifically that of the lung, head, and neck), respiratory disease, and accidents such as fires.
- Between 1992 and 1996, the American death toll from smoking exceeded the combined American death tolls of every war in U.S. history.
- Smoking stimulates the production of free radicals, which in turn hasten the aging process.
- An estimated 46,000 to 54,500 deaths occur annually from the effects of secondhand smoke.
- Infants and children exposed to cigarette smoke are far more likely to develop respiratory illnesses, including bronchitis, ear infections, and colds, and may be at increased risk of cancer.

Kicking the tobacco habit isn't easy; the majority of smokers try and fail repeatedly before they finally stop smoking for good. But as already noted, the reasons to stop far outnumber the reasons to continue. Here are a few tips to help you succeed:

- Set a date to quit—and stick with it. Concentrate on how good you will feel now that you are no longer smoking. Make a list of the health benefits and post it where you can see it often.
- Consult your physician regarding smoking cessation programs in your area, as well as cessation aids such as nicotine patches.

- Enlist a friend or coworker who is an ex-smoker to be on call to offer support when the cravings get too bad. It may also help to get a friend to quit with you.
- Remove all reminders of smoking from you house, including ashtrays, matches, and lighters. Ask family, friends, and coworkers to honor your decision by not smoking around you.
- In the beginning, try to avoid social situations in which you may be tempted to smoke.
- Satisfy oral cravings with low-cal candy, pretzels, or fruit and veggies. Squeeze a stress ball during times when you would normally have a cigarette in your hand.
- Get more exercise, even if it's just a walk around the block.
- Plan a nice reward for yourself after you've gone without a cigarette for a month. Use the money you would ordinarily have spent on cigarettes.
- Don't try to become a part-time or "social" smoker after you've quit. The vast majority of ex-smokers who have the "occasional" cigarette usually go back to being full-time smokers.
- Remember: Tobacco in any form is bad for you. That includes chewing tobacco and cigars.

FACTS

Here are a few more intriguing statistics:

- In 1900, only one in 100,000 Americans was 100 years or older. Today, the figure is estimated at one in 8,000.
- The number of centenarians is increasing at the rate of 8 percent per year in industrialized nations.
- If the current rate of growth continues, the United States will be home to nearly one million centenarians by the year 2050.
- Hallmark Cards, realizing an untapped market when it sees one, now offers cards for people celebrating their 100th birthday.

Cosmetic Surgery: What It Means to Your Anti-aging Regimen

For most people, anti-aging is a dual goal—feeling young while looking young. Living right can help you achieve the former, but sometimes we need some additional help with the latter. Toward that end, a growing number of men and women are having cosmetic surgery.

Studies show that slicing away the years via the surgeon's knife has never been more popular. Cosmetic surgery used to be a "woman thing," but doctors are reporting a dramatic increase in the number of male patients in our youth-obsessed society. The most popular procedures include face lifts, the removal of bags under the eyes, dermabrasion for the removal of small wrinkles, tummy tucks, and hair transplants for men.

In many cases, cosmetic surgery can, indeed, make a person look literally years younger. Yet many men and women spend thousands of dollars on procedures they really don't need, fearful that the smallest wrinkles make them look old. If you're contemplating cosmetic surgery, ask yourself the following questions:

- *Do you really need it?* If the bags under your eyes are so big they interfere with your vision, the answer is probably yes. But if your only signs of aging are a couple of facial wrinkles, you may want to reconsider. Are you doing this for yourself or because someone else says you need it?
- *Can you afford it?* Cosmetic surgery can run from several hundred to tens of thousands of dollars, depending on the complexity of the procedure. Insurance often pays for cosmetic surgery when it alleviates a specific health condition, but most purely cosmetic procedures are not covered.
- *Have you considered the risks?* No surgical procedure, regardless of simplicity, is 100 percent risk free. The most common complications associated with cosmetic surgery are infection and scarring. Make sure you fully understand all of the risks involved before agreeing to any cosmetic procedure.

If you genuinely want and need cosmetic surgery, do your homework before laying your money down. Check your doctor's credentials and reputation with your local medical society, and ask for references. If your doctor claims to be board certified in cosmetic surgery, contact the American Board of Medical Specialties for verification.

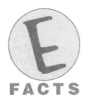

FACTS

Do you need a good excuse for going on vacation? A recent study of men at high risk for heart disease found that going on vacation may be more than just a frivolous pleasure; it may actually be good for your health. Researchers at the State University of New York at Oswego and the University of Pittsburgh analyzed data from a nine-year study of more than 12,000 men at high risk for coronary artery disease. The study participants had filled out questionnaires each year including a question about vacationing in the past twelve months. The conclusion: Those with regular annual vacations had a lower risk of death during the study period relative to those skipping their vacations.

CHAPTER 6
Related Diseases

One of the greatest hazards of aging is that it dramatically increases our risk of disease. With the exception of infection, trauma, genetic disorders, and certain youth-specific ailments, most disease is related to age. Most conditions are the result of age-related wear and tear on our body systems, though many conditions are caused or made worse by lifestyle and environment. We are going to take a close look at some of the most common age-related diseases and conditions in this chapter.

The Role of Genetics and Family History

More than 70 percent of aging can be associated in some way with our lifestyle and environment. As noted earlier, almost everything we do in life impacts on our health in one way or another, and over the years, these factors exert tremendous influence in how well we age and how long we live. Fortunately, much of this is under our control, and a concerted effort to maintain a healthful lifestyle can work wonders in counteracting the adverse effects of various external factors.

The remaining 30 percent of aging is associated with genetics and family history. Our genes define who we are and often predispose us to illness later in life. They also help determine how gracefully we age and how long we live.

Numerous studies have investigated the association between family history and the onset of certain medical conditions, but only a handful have actually looked at longevity trends between parents and their children. The 64 million dollar question in this handful of studies is, Does the fact that Mom and Dad lived to be 100 guarantee that their offspring will be similarly long lived, assuming they don't succumb to disease or injury?

The answer is surprising. The studies found an association between the longevity of parents and children, but it wasn't as strong as many had originally believed. The comprehensive Framingham Study, which has tracked more than 5,000 residents of Framingham, Massachusetts, since 1948, found only a 6 percent correlation between the age of the parents at the time of their deaths and the life span of their children. The study's conclusion: If your parents are long lived then your chances of living to a ripe old age are improved. But in the end, a great many other factors, such as familial risk of cancer or chronic disease, will play an equal or more important role in your longevity.

Let's look a bit closer at familial risk of disease, because it's important when analyzing longevity. Just because our parents lived to be 100 and didn't develop a genetically predisposed illness doesn't mean we're automatically out of the woods. We must also look at our grandparents, aunts, uncles, cousins, and siblings. Did they all live a long time in good health, or did cancer, heart disease, diabetes, or stroke afflict a noticeable percentage? The closer the family relationship, the more important their health and longevity in relation to our own. They, just as much as our parents, are indicators of what possibly lies ahead. The question remains, Is there anything we can do about it?

Common Diseases and Conditions of Aging
Stroke

This condition—in essence, a "brain attack"—results when blood flow to the brain is restricted due to clots or ruptured blood vessels in the brain. Without a steady blood flow, brain cells die from lack of oxygen. Stroke is the third leading killer in the United States, behind heart disease and cancer, and afflicts an estimated 500,000 Americans annually.

A severe stroke can result in instant death or debilitating physical problems, including total or partial paralysis, blindness, speech impairment, and cognitive dysfunction. The degree of disability depends on the type, severity, and location of the stroke and the timing of treatment. The effects of strokes caused by clots (known as ischemic strokes) can often be minimized with the rapid infusion of clot-destroying drugs. There is no known treatment for strokes caused by ruptured blood vessels (known as hemorrhagic strokes).

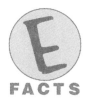
FACTS

Vacations may protect health by reducing stress, which is a known risk factor for many diseases. Vacations may also work their magic by providing opportunities to engage in restorative behaviors such as exercise and interactions with family and friends.

Stroke is definitely an age-related disorder; incidence increases dramatically after age fifty-five. The most common type seen among the elderly is ischemic stroke, which is typically associated with atherosclerosis.

Dementia

Dementia is a common brain disorder among the elderly and is generally defined as an observable, irreversible decline in mental abilities.

In years past, the many different forms of dementia were grouped under the umbrella term "senility," but doctors now know that dementia comes in many forms and from an intriguing variety of causes.

Dementia is generally viewed as irreversible, though there are some potentially reversible causes, including drug side effects, emotional disorders, metabolic or endocrine disorders, nutritional deficiencies, arteriosclerotic complications, and certain types of brain tumors.

Most forms of dementia are progressive, meaning they worsen over time, and result in an array of functional impairment. People with severe dementia, for example, typically lose all memory (with long-term memory usually being the last to go) and are almost always unable to clothe, feed, or bathe themselves. They require full-time care and are dependent on others for virtually all of their physical needs.

Doctors divide the many types of dementia into two categories: cortical and subcortical. Alzheimer's disease (which we'll be discussing shortly) is a classic form of cortical dementia; examples of subcortical dementia include those resulting from Huntington's disease, multiple sclerosis, AIDS, and hydrocephalus.

Individuals with cortical dementia typically experience more severe memory impairment than those with subcortical dementia. They also tend to have a poor response to verbal cues and greater language impairment, among other symptoms.

Heart Disease

Despite advances in diagnosis, treatment, and prevention, heart disease remains the nation's number one killer, accounting for nearly 940,000 deaths every year—the majority of them among people fifty and older. The economic cost of heart disease is equally high: more than $108 billion a year for treatment, lost work time, and so forth.

According to the American Heart Association, men have a 42 percent chance of developing heart disease over the course of their lives. But women are also at risk, particularly after menopause, when the risk of cardiovascular disease actually exceeds that of men. An estimated 250,000 women over age sixty die from heart attacks each year—six times that of breast cancer, which tends to garner much more publicity.

Many heart attacks are the result of atherosclerosis, or "clogged arteries." Atherosclerosis results from an accumulation of fatty cholesterol deposits known as plaque. Over time, this buildup greatly reduces blood flow to various parts of the body, forcing the heart to work harder and harder until it finally gives out. Other contributors to heart disease include high blood pressure and diabetes. Lifestyle factors such as years of smoking, obesity, and a lack of physical activity can also increase your risk.

Cancer

Cancer results when previously healthy cells begin to mutate and grow out of control. Left unchecked, cancer cells can develop into tumors that leech vital nutrients from neighboring cells and organs. Cancerous cells can also travel throughout the body via the blood or lymphatic system, affecting other organs in a process known medically as metastasis.

All cells have the potential to become cancerous. The body's immune system is able to handle the occasional "rogue" cell. However, problems result when cancerous growth exceeds the body's ability to keep it in check.

Cancer can be divided into five basic types: carcinoma, sarcoma, myeloma, lymphoma, and leukemia. The most common type of cancer is carcinoma, which often affects the skin, bowel, lungs, and certain hormone-sensitive organs such as the breast and prostate. Most doctors agree that nearly all men will develop some form of prostate cancer if they live long enough. However, prostate cancer tends to be very slow growing, and the majority of patients die from other causes. The most deadly type of cancer is sarcoma, which typically develops in the connective and muscle tissues. Fortunately, sarcoma is also relatively rare, as is myeloma, which initially forms in the plasma cells and destroys bone marrow.

Cancer is the second biggest killer in the United States, just behind heart disease. It can affect people of any age, but our risk increases dramatically with age. Risk factors are many, but diet apparently plays a significant role in the formation of many types of cancer. In fact, after decades of study, the National Cancer Institute now estimates that 35 percent of cancer deaths are related to certain elements in the foods we eat. At the same time, the right kind of diet also appears quite effective in preventing many types of cancer.

Arthritis

This extremely common disorder is probably more closely associated with old age than any other ailment. It afflicts one in seven Americans to some degree and, as the baby boomer generation ages, will probably become epidemic in coming years, according to the Arthritis Foundation.

There are more than 100 different types of arthritis. The most common form is osteoarthritis, which generally involves a breakdown of cartilage in one or more joints, followed by rheumatoid arthritis, which is characterized by an inflammation of the joint membrane. Less common forms of arthritis include ankylosing spondylitis (an inflammation of ligaments attached to the bone), lupus (a connective tissue disease), and gout (characterized by deposits of uric acid crystals in the joint fluid). The most common symptoms of osteoarthritis are pain, swelling, stiffness, and loss of motion.

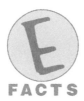

FACTS

A common cause of low testosterone levels is a condition known as hypogonadism, which can be caused by an injury or infection in the testicles, a chromosomal disorder known as Klinefelter's syndrome, and diseases of the hypothalamus and pituitary gland. The most common symptoms include loss of libido, fatigue, mood swings, dry skin, aching joints, osteoporosis, and weight loss. Many doctors believe that some of the common symptoms of aging seen in older men may actually be the result of hypogonadism. In fact, some specialists estimate that as many as 20 percent of men over fifty may have the disorder and could be helped with testosterone supplements.

There is no known prevention for osteoarthritis, though maintaining an ideal body weight and good muscle tone may reduce trauma to the joints. The pain and inflammation of arthritis is typically treated with topical heating gels and oral analgesics such as acetaminophen, or anti-inflammatories such as ibuprofen. The treatment of arthritis is a multimillion dollar industry, and new therapies are being developed all the time.

Osteoporosis

This condition is characterized by a loss of bone density and strength and afflicts more than 25 million Americans, more than 80 percent of them female. Because of the toll it takes on the skeletal system, osteoporosis is the primary underlying cause of bone fractures in postmenopausal women and the elderly. The most common sites for osteoporosis-related fractures are the spinal column, the wrist, and the hip. In severe cases, incapacitating fractures can result from minor falls and the simplest of acts, such as bending over.

Hip fractures in the elderly are now one of the most serious health problems in the United States. In fact, they are associated with more deaths, more disability, and higher medical costs than all other osteoporosis-related fractures combined. The results can be tragic: Up to 20 percent of elderly adults die within a year of fracturing their hips, and fewer than half of the survivors are able to return to full activity.

Age is one of the biggest risk factors for osteoporosis, followed closely by gender. For example, osteoporosis is six to eight times more common in women than men because lower estrogen levels following menopause cause women to lose bone mass more rapidly. Other risk factors include early menopause, ethnic background (Asian and Caucasian women are at greater risk than African-American women), lack of weight-bearing exercise, inadequate calcium consumption over one's lifetime, body weight (thin, small-boned women, particularly athletes, whose menstrual periods have stopped from overexercising), heredity, smoking, and alcohol consumption.

Diabetes

Most people tend to think of diabetes as a relatively benign chronic condition that's easily treated with insulin. However, the facts say otherwise. According to the American Diabetes Association, the disease is the fourth leading cause of death in the United States, claiming 160,000 lives each year. It also carries a huge financial burden; treatment costs and lost work time are estimated at nearly $100 billion annually.

However, all is not lost for diabetes patients. The ten-year Diabetes Control and Complications Trial (DCCT) concluded that a tightly controlled and managed treatment plan can reduce the risk of long-term complications by 50 percent or more.

There are two forms of diabetes: insulin-dependent and non-insulin-dependent. With insulin-dependent, or Type I, diabetes, which is most commonly seen in children and young adults, the pancreas fails to produce enough insulin to properly regulate blood sugar levels. With non-insulin-dependent, or Type II, diabetes, which more commonly afflicts the middle-aged and elderly, the pancreas still produces insulin, but the body requires more than is being produced, or does not respond properly to it. This phenomenon is known medically as insulin resistance.

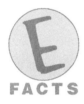

FACTS

The medical profession is filled with a wide variety of physicians and specialties. It's difficult to choose a doctor if you don't understand what each specialty does.

- Family practitioners specialize in family medicine and provide care for people of all ages.
- General practitioners specialize in general medicine.
- Pediatricians specialize in providing care for children under age eighteen.
- Gynecologists specialize in treating female problems and may also provide primary care for the special needs of women.
- Geriatricians are specialists who treat people over age sixty-five and may also provide primary care.

Without sufficient amounts of insulin, blood sugar levels can climb to dangerous levels. As a result, the body's energy level drops and you feel tired and listless. Fatigue is one of the most common symptoms of diabetes, along with frequent urination, abnormal thirst, and sudden, unexplained weight loss. Related complications include reduced circulation to the lower limbs (often resulting in the amputation of toes and feet), nervous system damage, kidney failure, blindness, and heart disease.

Researchers know more now than ever before about diabetes, but they are still uncertain as to its exact cause. Insulin-dependent diabetes may be the result of an autoimmune reaction in which the body attacks its own tissues as if they were foreign proteins. Non-insulin-dependent diabetes is most likely a genetic flaw, though other factors may also play a role, including poor diet and obesity (more than 80 percent of non-insulin-dependent diabetics are very overweight).

Aging on the Brain

Despite being so well protected behind the thick bone of the cranium, the brain can experience a wide variety of problems and disorders, especially in old age. Some of these conditions, such as stroke and Alzheimer's disease, are physical in nature; others are the result of environmental factors, such as lead poisoning or exposure to pesticides.

Some brain disorders, such as Alzheimer's disease, simply occur, and there's nothing we can do about it. However, other disorders, such as strokes, often can be prevented through a healthful lifestyle, controlling blood pressure, and by taking certain precautions, such as a daily aspirin tablet to reduce the risk of clots. Lifestyle abuses such as lifelong smoking, excessive alcohol consumption, and the use of certain illicit drugs, can also result in brain disorders. Following is a review of the most common brain disorders with advice, where appropriate, on what we can do to prevent them.

Stroke

Stroke is a medical condition characterized by sudden or gradual neurological impairment resulting from reduced blood flow to the brain and the subsequent death of brain cells, which are dependent on blood for oxygen. Brain cells are very sensitive and begin to starve when deprived of oxygen for even a few minutes. Prolonged oxygen deprivation usually results in permanent brain damage.

Commonly referred to as a "brain attack," stroke is the third leading cause of death in the United States, behind heart disease and cancer. An estimated 500,000 Americans experience a new or recurrent stroke every year, and nearly a third of cases are fatal. According to the American Heart Association, stroke is the leading cause of serious disability in the United States and is responsible for nearly $40 billion in health care costs and lost productivity annually.

Risk of stroke increases dramatically after age fifty-five. Common risk factors include poorly managed hypertension (high blood pressure), a family history of stroke, a personal history of "mini-strokes," known as transient ischemic attacks (TIAs), atherosclerosis (particularly in the neck, heart, and legs), atrial fibrillation, and a history of smoking.

The Effects of a Stroke

The effects of a stroke vary dramatically and can range from loss of a particular sense such as vision or speech to memory loss, partial or complete paralysis, and even death. Some effects of a stroke may disappear over time; others can be treated with physical therapy. However, some effects worsen over time. The extent of damage resulting from a stroke depends on the severity of the attack, where in the brain it occurs, and how quickly the patient receives medical attention. Very often damage can be minimized with the rapid administration of clot-busting drugs.

Doctors divide stroke into two main categories: ischemic and hemorrhagic. Ischemic strokes are the most common, accounting for nearly 80 percent of all stroke events, and occur when an artery delivering blood to the brain becomes blocked. The primary villain in this scenario is atherosclerosis, a process which slowly clogs arterial inner walls with fatty deposits until only a trickle of blood can get through.

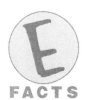

FACTS

Age affects our metabolism in a number of ways. One of the most problematic is a reduced ability to absorb and metabolize drugs, which can adversely affect their efficacy. Worse, the majority of older people take more than one medication, increasing the risk of side effects or dangerous interactions.

Atherosclerosis does not actually cause ischemic strokes, but it sets in play the conditions that make a stroke much more likely. The real obstruction that cuts off blood flow in an ischemic stroke is a blood clot, which often develops through a process known as thrombosis. Clots are more likely to form at the site of a fatty blockage because the deposit causes blood to flow in a turbulent fashion. This turbulence stimulates blood to clot just as it does when we cut our finger. When a blood clot develops at the site of an atherosclerotic formation, it usually blocks blood flow to part of the brain, resulting in a stroke.

Ischemic stroke can also be caused by a traveling blood clot, for example, one that originally forms in one of the heart's chambers. The clot travels through the bloodstream until it reaches a vessel too small to let it continue (very often one that is clogged with fatty deposits). Like a tiny dam, it blocks the vessel and halts blood flow at that point.

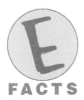

FACTS

According to the Centers for Disease Control and Prevention, the number of people with arthritis will increase 57 percent by the year 2020, and the number of people with arthritis-related activity limitation will increase by a startling 66 percent.

Sometimes a transient ischemic attack (TIA), or "mini-stroke," will occur shortly before a full-blown ischemic stroke. The results are stroke-like symptoms lasting anywhere from five minutes to twenty-four hours. TIAs commonly occur when a blood clot develops at the site of an atherosclerotic deposit but quickly dissolves, or an embolism gets stuck in a narrowed vessel but is eventually dislodged. A transient ischemic attack can also be the result of a blockage by itself. In most such cases, the atherosclerotic deposit restricts blood flow to the point where the brain no longer receives sufficient oxygen. Brain cells seldom die as a result of a TIA, and recovery is usually very quick.

The remaining 20 percent of strokes are typically of the hemorrhagic variety and occur when weakened blood vessels within the brain burst and bleed into the surrounding tissue. The escaped blood can press on nearby blood vessels, cutting off blood flow and depriving surrounding tissue of oxygen. Though more rare than ischemic strokes, hemorrhagic strokes tend to be more serious and affect a larger portion of the brain. The symptoms are usually more sudden and severe, and hemorrhagic strokes result in a greater number of deaths.

One of the most common causes of a hemorrhagic stroke is an aneurysm, which occurs when the wall of a blood vessel weakens and bulges outward like a squeezed balloon. Left untreated, an aneurysm will continue to weaken over time, increasing the risk of a rupture. Aneurysms are much more likely to rupture in patients with elevated blood pressure. A hemorrhagic stroke can also result from an arteriovenous malformation, which is a cluster of weakened blood vessels that usually forms during fetal development or at birth. These malformed vessels start out structurally weak and are prone to bursting from the normal forces of healthy blood flow. Taking blood thinners like aspirin may worsen hemorrhagic strokes.

Stroke Symptoms

Because the effects of a stroke often can be minimized with prompt treatment, it's important that everyone be aware of the following most common stroke symptoms:

- Sudden weakness or numbness on one side of the face, one arm, or one leg.
- Sudden dimness or loss of vision, particularly in one eye.
- Sudden, severe headache.
- Sudden inability to speak, or trouble understanding speech.
- Sudden, unexplained dizziness, unsteadiness, or falls.

Anyone experiencing any of these symptoms should seek immediate medical attention, especially if the symptoms worsen over the next hour.

It's the rare stroke patient that comes away from the experience without at least some lasting physical or mental effects, including one or more impaired senses, impaired mobility, or memory loss. Side effects are based on where in the brain the stroke occurred and the severity of the event. Even with prompt treatment, some minimal effects may remain as a result of site-specific brain damage. But as noted earlier, many of these effects can be at least partially alleviated with physical or occupational therapy.

It should be noted that psychological problems are a common side effect of a stroke. Some mood changes may be the result of the stroke itself, though it's more common for stroke victims to become depressed, angry, or frustrated as a result of their new physical limitations. This is particularly true among people who were very active before the stroke event but now find themselves unable to perform the simplest activity. Family members and friends should be aware of these potential personality changes and do what they can to assist the stroke patient in his or her recovery and rehabilitation.

An accurate diagnosis of stroke is important because other situations can mimic stroke symptoms, including brain tumors, a drug overdose, and certain types of infection. A variety of imaging techniques, including magnetic resonance imaging (MRI), X-ray angioplasty, and computed tomography (also known as a CT scan), are commonly used to diagnose a stroke and rule out other possible causes. Computed tomography is especially useful because it can quickly confirm that a stroke is in progress, tell the doctor whether it is an ischemic stroke or a hemorrhagic stroke, and detail the extent of brain damage.

Treatment of stroke depends on what kind it is and the severity of the event. In the case of ischemic stroke, the primary goal of treatment is to eliminate the blockage, improve blood flow to the brain, and take whatever steps necessary to prevent complications. One of the most effective weapons in the treatment of ischemic stroke is clot-busting drugs such as tissue plasminogen activator (t-PA), which quickly dissolves blood clots at the site. The sooner such drugs are administered, the more effective they are and the lower the potential for stroke-related side effects. Most thrombolytic agents work best when administered within three hours of the onset of stroke symptoms.

Once the stroke has been stopped and the patient has been stabilized, the long journey to recovery begins. Depending on the type and severity of residual physical and mental complications, rehabilitation can take weeks, months, and even years. For example, if partial paralysis is involved, the patient must learn to walk and function all over again.

This can be a very trying time for the patient and his family, and strong social support is extremely important in maintaining a positive attitude.

Many complications of stroke may seem overwhelming at first but gradually lessen in severity as an unaffected portion of the brain takes over those particular functions. Physical therapy can also help stroke patients learn to cope with physical limitations, often to the point of near normal function.

Stroke Prevention

Stroke prevention should be a priority for everyone, but particularly for people fifty-five and older. One of the best ways to reduce your risk of stroke is to live a healthful lifestyle. By eating right, exercising regularly, and avoiding harmful habits such as smoking and excessive alcohol consumption, you can greatly diminish many of the known risk factors, such as hypertension and high cholesterol levels.

Smoking is an extremely hazardous habit for people at high risk of stroke because certain chemicals found in cigarette smoke can affect the blood in such a way that it's more prone to clotting. In addition, nicotine damages the interior walls of blood vessels and makes them more susceptible to atherosclerosis.

Individuals at risk of ischemic stroke, including those with known blood vessel abnormalities or those who have had a transient ischemic attack or a previous stroke, should be aware that there are a number of ways to prevent the occurrence of a first or second stroke. For example, blood flow can often be maximized through a narrowed vessel via surgery. One common treatment is carotid endarterectomy, which is the surgical removal of fatty deposits in a diseased carotid artery. By removing the atherosclerotic deposit, blood flow to the brain is greatly improved, and the risk of a stroke-inducing blood clot is diminished.

Anticoagulant drugs, also known as blood thinners, can help prevent an ischemic stroke by making it more difficult for blood to clot. Common aspirin can also be used as an anticoagulant. This is why many doctors encourage their older patients, or those otherwise at risk, to take a single aspirin tablet several times a week.

Dementia

There are many forms of dementia, almost all of which afflict older populations, but the most common type is Alzheimer's disease. Most forms of dementia are progressive and result in gradual functional impairment, including the development of multiple cognitive deficits. The most common include memory loss, language disturbances, impaired motor function, and a loss of abstract thinking ability.

The most commonly seen forms of dementia are organic in origin, meaning they simply develop as a natural part of aging. However, some forms of cognitive deficit are known to have outside causes, including drug interactions, metabolic or endocrine disorders, poor nutrition, infections, and brain tumors or trauma. When detected early, many of these problems can be successfully cured, with a complete reversal of symptoms.

The symptoms of dementia can vary depending on type and cause but generally include increasing memory loss (with short-term memory typically the first to be affected), "dropping" words (difficulty coming up with the right word at the right time), a distorted sense of time (the passage of days often seems like weeks), increasing difficulty performing high-brain functions such as balancing a checkbook or making change, and noticeable changes in personality, including increased irritability, anger, and frustration.

Because dementia tends to progress slowly, it may take months and even years before the condition is noticeable to the patient and his loved ones. The occasional "senior moment" becomes increasingly frequent until medical care is finally sought. That's when an umbrella diagnosis of dementia may be made, though it is often difficult to determine the exact type and cause. A differential diagnosis—one in which all possible disorders are eliminated until the correct one is determined—is often used to identify Alzheimer's disease, though an absolute diagnosis is impossible until after death, when a brain biopsy can be performed.

Researchers are working hard to find out how and why dementia occurs. At the moment, there is no cure for most age-related forms of the condition, though a handful of prescriptions drugs are available that have shown great effectiveness in slowing many of the most common symptoms, particularly memory loss, when taken during the early stages. One of the primary goals of ongoing research into dementia is the development of some type of vaccine or other preventative measure, but such a wonder drug is years away.

The cost of dementia is tremendous, both financially and emotionally. As the condition grows worse, most dementia patients require round-the-clock care, either in an institution, such as a nursing home, or by at-home caregivers. Many families choose to care for demented loved ones at home rather than place them in a nursing home, and the resulting stress can take a heavy toll on all involved. In addition, paying for in-home support can deplete financial resources at a startling rate, since government assistance can be difficult to obtain. Some families, stressed to the breaking point, have been known to "dump" loved ones in hospital emergency rooms because they simply couldn't take it anymore.

As medical research extends the boundaries of longevity, how society deals with the problem of dementia will become increasingly important. Because we're living longer, more and more people will develop the condition in its varied forms in coming years, requiring expensive, long-term care. It's an issue that is sure to affect the majority of Americans in some way within the next decade.

Alzheimer's Disease

Alzheimer's disease is by far the most common type of age-related dementia in the world. This debilitating disorder can have a huge impact on the lives of those afflicted, as well as loved ones, friends, and caregivers, but the more you know about it, the better you can cope with its consequences. Research into the causes of Alzheimer's disease and potential treatments or cures is ongoing, with promising findings occurring all the time. In the not too distant future, a vaccine or pill may be discovered that will prevent Alzheimer's disease and increase overall brain longevity.

Alzheimer's disease was first described, by German psychiatrist Alois Alzheimer, in 1906. At that time, the condition was considered relatively rare and believed to affect only young people. As a result, it was initially referred to as presenile dementia.

Today, late-onset Alzheimer's disease is known to be the most common cause of loss of mental function in people over sixty-five. Approximately 4 million Americans are believed to have Alzheimer's disease, 90 percent of them over age sixty.

The indicators of Alzheimer's disease are fairly clear cut, though an absolute diagnosis is impossible until after death. In general, the brains of Alzheimer's patients contain distinctive, abnormally shaped proteins known as tangles and plaques. Tangles are long, silklike tendrils found inside neurons. Plaques are clumps of silklike fibers that typically form outside the neurons in adjacent brain tissue. The areas most commonly afflicted by tangles and plaques are related to memory.

In the 1980s, researchers found that a compound in plaques, known as amyloid protein, may actually be poisonous to brain cells. And more recent research suggests that a protein called tau may be responsible for the telltale tangles found in the brains of Alzheimer's patients. In healthy brains, tau gives neurons structural support, but in Alzheimer's patients, this structural support collapses into useless twists and tangles.

Signs and Symptoms of Alzheimer's

Memory loss is the most common indication of Alzheimer's disease, but it is not the only one. According to the Alzheimer's Association, people with the disease also experience a noticeable decline in cognitive function and changes in behavior. Following are ten common symptoms of Alzheimer's disease:

- *Memory loss that affects job skills.* Occasionally forgetting an assignment or deadline is normal and nothing to worry about, but frequent forgetfulness or confusion at work could signal that something is wrong.
- *Difficulty performing familiar tasks.* It's easy to get distracted when performing an everyday task, but the problem is far more serious for someone with Alzheimer's disease. While you might forget that you had put a pot on to boil for tea, a victim of Alzheimer's disease will also forget what the boiling pot was for.
- *Problems with language.* We're all prone to a slip of the tongue now and then, but people with Alzheimer's disease often forget the most

simple of words, or use words inappropriately, making them difficult to understand.

- *Disorientation to time and place.* Everyone has walked into a room and completely forgotten why they were there, or stood in the middle of the grocery store trying to remember what they needed to buy. However, people with Alzheimer's disease often become lost on their own street, confused about where they are, and unable to find their way home.

- *Poor or decreased judgment.* This includes wearing clothes inappropriate for the climate (such as several sweaters on a hot day) or the location (such as a bathrobe while grocery shopping).

- *Problems with abstract thinking.* Not everyone is a whiz at math, but the problem can be much worse for someone with Alzheimer's disease because of an inability to recognize numbers or perform basic calculations.

- *Misplacing things.* We've all misplaced our keys at one time or another, but people with Alzheimer's disease often place items in very inappropriate places. For example, they might put a purse in the oven and then forget how it got there.

- *Changes in mood or behavior.* Healthy people go through a wide variety of moods and emotions each day, but these changes tend to be much more rapid in people with Alzheimer's disease.

- *Changes in personality.* Personality tends to change somewhat with age, but such changes are usually more dramatic and uncharacteristic in people with Alzheimer's disease. For example, someone who has been friendly and outgoing their entire life may become suspicious or fearful as a result of the disease.

- *Loss of initiative.* Everyone gets tired of housework or business activities, but most people retain and eventually regain their interest. Someone with Alzheimer's disease may remain uninterested and unmotivated in most if not all of his or her usual pursuits.

It's important to note that the typical symptoms of Alzheimer's disease are very gradual in their onset. During the early stages of the disease, Alzheimer's patients experience relatively mild problems learning new information and remembering to perform routine tasks such as locking the front door when they leave for work. Episodes of forgetfulness may be laughed off or attributed to old age.

Over time, however, Alzheimer's patients begin to have trouble recalling recent events and finding the right words to express themselves. Memory lapses become increasingly common as the disease progresses, with short-term memory failing first. For example, many Alzheimer's patients can tell you everyone they went to high school with but not what they had for lunch a half hour ago. As the disease worsens, the patient may begin wandering, only to find that they can't remember how to get home again.

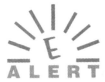

Water is essential for good health, but too much water can be deadly. As amazing as it seems, a small percentage of people actually become addicted to water and drink it to the point of intoxication. Excessive water consumption can make a person intoxicated by altering the body's sodium level, but the risks are high. Too much water can actually cause a heart attack, seizures, coma, and death from swelling of the brain.

Personality changes become more evident, including increasing irritability or withdrawal as the patient tries to come to grips with what's happening. The realization that one may have Alzheimer's disease can be frightening and frustrating, leading to depression and other problems.

During the later stages of the disease, the Alzheimer's patient becomes increasingly unable to care for himself or herself. The patient may become delusional, need help dressing, and forget to eat unless reminded. He or she may also need help with bathing and using the bathroom. Eventually, the patient will become completely incapacitated and will require round-the-clock care.

Alzheimer's patients can live with the disease for several years and usually die from related complications such as pneumonia, or general wasting away as they take in less and less nourishment. In general, the time between initial diagnosis and death is seven to ten years, though every case is unique. Some people succumb to complications more quickly;

others linger far longer. Contributing factors include the age of onset, other medical problems the patient may have, and the care he or she receives.

The Causes of Alzheimer's Disease

Despite years of research, Alzheimer's disease remains a medical mystery. Doctors still don't know what causes the disease, though they have determined that certain groups are more at risk of developing it than others. People with a family history of Alzheimer's disease, for example, are more likely to become afflicted than those with no family history.

Because of this fact, researchers are putting a greater focus on genetics to see if they can shed more light on the causes of Alzheimer's disease and possible cures or preventions. One intriguing study found that people with a specific version of the apolipoprotein E gene are several times more likely to develop Alzheimer's disease than carriers of other forms of the apoE gene. The most common version of this gene in the general public is apoE3. Almost half of all late-onset Alzheimer's patients have the less common apoE4 version, and studies suggest that this gene plays an integral role in the disease. Perhaps in the future, gene therapy will allow doctors to "turn off" the apoE4 gene, thus reducing risk of Alzheimer's disease for a large segment of the population.

A number of early studies suggested that environmental factors may also play a role in the development of Alzheimer's disease. Aluminum, for example, has long been considered a culprit, and many people have thrown away aluminum cooking pots for fear that the metal could put them at risk. However, studies into the role of aluminum have shown mixed results at best. Some studies detected high levels of the metal in Alzheimer's patients; others found relatively low levels. Studies into other potential causes such as zinc exposure and food borne poisons have also yielded inconclusive results.

Diagnosing Alzheimer's Disease

As noted, a definitive diagnosis of Alzheimer's disease can only be done by examining brain tissue under a microscope to detect telltale plaques and tangles. However, doctors are able to diagnose the condition with relative accuracy using a variety of other techniques that gauge physical and cognitive changes common to Alzheimer's disease. A recently developed urine test for isoprostane seems to correlate well with Alzheimer's disease and may play a useful role in screening for Alzheimer's disease.

Foremost, however, doctors want to rule out other conditions that may be mimicking the symptoms of Alzheimer's disease, such as a stroke, drug interaction, or a brain tumor. This involves a thorough physical examination, including special brain scans. Next, the patient may be given a neuropsychological examination designed to evaluate his or her ability to perform specific mental tasks. This test is relatively easy for someone without dementia but can be difficult for someone with failing cognitive function. A family medical history may also be taken to determine if any family members were stricken with Alzheimer's disease.

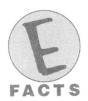

FACTS

The reproduction of DNA within our cells is vital to our survival, and natural repair systems quickly leap into action when errors are made. Be thankful that they do, because if these repair processes did not exist, researchers believe that within just one year, sufficient damage would accumulate in our cells to make them stop working entirely.

Early diagnosis is important because it may improve chances of benefiting from existing treatments, maximize quality time with loved ones, and relieve anxiety. Early diagnosis may also identify the problem not as Alzheimer's disease but as a form of reversible dementia.

Treatment of Alzheimer's Disease

Right now there is no cure for Alzheimer's disease. The best doctors can do is treat its symptoms and try to slow its progression with medication. The Food and Drug Administration has approved a handful of drugs that increase or improve the function of acetylcholine, a neurotransmitter known to affect memory, and other drug treatments are under investigation.

Researchers are also studying the fact that Alzheimer's patients often experience inflammation in the brain, which could be associated with the production of amyloid, the protein responsible for plaques. One theory speculates that anti-inflammatory drugs may help prevent this inflammation, dramatically slowing the progression of the disease.

Until a cure for Alzheimer's disease can be found, medication and nonpharmacological treatments are often used to help alleviate some of the common behavioral problems associated with the disease, such as agitation, aggression, insomnia, and wandering. Nonpharmacological approaches include family education and counseling (to learn how to better cope with the behaviors of a loved one with Alzheimer's disease), environment modification (many disturbing behaviors are triggered by color, light, and noise), and planning activities that help the Alzheimer's patient focus on pleasurable or useful tasks.

A variety of drug treatments can be used to help quell certain behaviors when nonpharmacological approaches don't work. Drugs commonly used to treat behavioral symptoms such as agitation, paranoia, delusions, or depression include antipsychotics, anxiolytics, and antidepressants.

Caring for the Alzheimer's Patient

Alzheimer's disease can be a devastating disorder, both for patients and for their loved ones. It is an insidious condition that progresses with damning slowness, giving everyone involved plenty of time to ponder the future with fear and uncertainty. Education helps, but no one is really prepared to deal with Alzheimer's disease when it reaches the later stages.

Family members and friends should do all they can to comfort and reassure the Alzheimer's patient who, during lucid moments, may be overcome with frustration, anxiety, and depression. It's difficult to know that your memory is gradually eroding and that there is nothing you can do about it. Strong social support is vital during these times.

The treatment of Alzheimer's disease and its symptoms should be aggressive, but eventually the disease will have completely devastated the patient's mind to the point where he or she is no longer the person he or she once was. This can be difficult for family members to accept. If the burden becomes too much, loved ones are encouraged to talk with their clergy or join an Alzheimer's support group; it often helps to talk with others who share similar experiences.

As the disease progresses, patients will require more and more attention until their care becomes a full-time job. Many family members try to care for their stricken loved ones alone, unwilling to consider institutional care. This is understandable, but you shouldn't feel guilty about seeking outside help. No one can function in this way twenty-four hours a day, seven days a week, without experiencing health problems of his or her own. Be wary of caregiver burnout and do what you must to take care of your own needs. At the very least, hire someone to watch your loved one a few hours each day so that you can get away and have some time to yourself.

Heart Disease

As noted earlier, heart disease in its many forms is the number one killer in the United States. It is also one of the most preventable age-related medical conditions; risk can be dramatically reduced through regular exercise and a moderately healthy diet. Unfortunately, most heart patients don't realize that until it's too late.

In developed nations, cardiovascular disease is the most common cause of death and hospitalization in the elderly, and coronary atherosclerosis is the most common underlying cause. Studies on cadavers have shown that 65 to 75 percent of men aged fifty to eighty years and 60 to 65 percent of women aged seventy to eighty years have significantly blocked arteries, yet less than half this number show symptoms of coronary disease. The incidence and severity of coronary atherosclerosis increase so rapidly with age that more than half of all deaths in people aged sixty-five years and older are due to coronary disease, and about three-fourths of all deaths from ischemic heart disease occur in the elderly.

Coronary Heart Disease

The most common symptom of coronary heart disease is angina pectoris, a squeezing chest pain that usually radiates to the neck, jaw, back, and left arm. This is a signal that blood flow to the heart muscle is insufficient when extra work is required from the heart muscle. Angina is typically triggered by exercise or other physical exertion, or by strong emotions such as anger or fear. Coronary heart disease can also lead to a heart attack, which usually occurs when a blood clot forms at the site of an arterial blockage and inhibits or completely stops the flow of blood to a section of the heart. When a heart attack (known medically as a cardiac infarction) occurs, part of the heart muscle is deprived of oxygen and dies. This also causes the crushing chest pain that is a common symptom of a heart attack. Other symptoms of a heart attack include nausea, vomiting, and profuse sweating. An estimated one-third of heart attacks are fatal, though most patients can be saved if they receive immediate medical treatment. This is why everyone should know the symptoms of a heart attack and act on them quickly.

There are numerous risk factors for coronary heart disease, including smoking, lack of exercise, diabetes, hypertension, and obesity. The most telling factor, however, is an elevated level of cholesterol in the bloodstream, which most commonly results from a diet of fatty, high-cholesterol foods. (Some genetic disorders can also cause high blood-cholesterol levels.)

Doctors used to believe that coronary heart disease was primarily a male disorder, but new research has proved this to be a myth. The disorder afflicts men and women equally, though women tend to develop the disease later in life than men do.

There is no cure for coronary heart disease, though it often can be controlled with medication (particularly cholesterol-lowering drugs such as lovastatin, simvastatin, or pravastatin) and changes in lifestyle. The most common recommendations made by doctors are to exercise more and to eat fewer high-fat foods and more fruit and vegetables. And, of course, smoking is strongly discouraged.

Angina pectoris, one of the most common symptoms of coronary heart disease, can be relieved through a variety of medications. Nitroglycerin has been the drug of choice for decades, though many patients now find relief through beta blockers and calcium channel blockers. Angina patients may also be encouraged to take an aspirin tablet every day to prevent the formation of blood clots. (Aspirin works by interfering with the clotting ability of platelets.)

In cases in which lifestyle changes and medication are ineffective in relieving coronary heart disease, patients may need to undergo coronary bypass surgery. As its name suggests, the procedure involves removing a length of artery from elsewhere in the body and literally bypassing the blockage by attaching one end of the artery to the aorta and the other end to the coronary artery. Increasingly, surgeons use an artery from the inside of the chest wall because bypasses created this way tend to be extremely durable, reducing the need for a second bypass.

An alternative to coronary bypass surgery is percutaneous transluminal coronary angioplasty, more commonly known as balloon angioplasty. In this procedure, a deflated balloon is passed through the patient's coronary arteries to the site of a blockage, then inflated. This crushes the plaque against the arterial wall and restores normal blood flow through the artery.

Coronary heart disease is easier to prevent than it is to treat, especially if you have a family history of heart problems. The keys to keeping coronary heart disease at bay are regular, heart-strengthening exercise (at least four times a week) and maintaining a healthful diet that is low in fat and cholesterol and high in antioxidant-rich fruits and vegetables. It's also a good idea to avoid stress as much as possible, and to see your doctor annually for a checkup. Most importantly, seek medical attention immediately at the first sign of a heart attack. Rapid treatment can dramatically reduce your risk of long-term complications.

Other Forms of Heart Disease

Coronary heart disease is the type of heart disease most people are familiar with. However, this is just one form of heart disease that can develop as we age. In fact, there are several other types that can have an adverse affect on our health and, therefore, our longevity.

Myocarditis

This condition is an inflammation of the heart muscle. In the past, it was commonly caused by rheumatic fever; today, the most common cause is a viral infection. Most cases of myocarditis go away on their own, though some people experience repeated episodes, which can lead to permanent damage of the heart muscle. The result can be a reduction in the heart's ability to pump blood efficiently and an increased risk of developing abnormal rhythms.

Cardiomyopathy

This is an umbrella term for any condition that damages and weakens the heart muscle. Causes range from a viral infection to rheumatic fever, a vitamin deficiency, thyroid problems, and a genetic disorder known as hemochromatosis, which is characterized by a buildup of iron in the heart muscle cells. Depending on the cause, cardiomyopathy can often be controlled with medication. But severe cases can lead to progressive weakening of the heart muscle and even heart failure.

Pericarditis

This condition is an inflammation of the sac that surrounds the heart. It is typically caused by a viral infection but may also result from arthritis or an autoimmune disease such as lupus. Pericarditis can also be a complication of late-stage kidney disease, lymphoma, or lung cancer, or a side effect of radiation therapy or certain drugs. The condition often disappears on its own, though it can be treated with anti-inflammatory drugs. Fortunately, pericarditis rarely results in permanent damage to the heart muscle.

Endocarditis

This condition is an infection of the inner lining of the heart, though the damage is usually to the heart valves. Endocarditis most often develops when bacteria from somewhere else in the body enter the bloodstream and begin to grow on the flaps of one of the heart valves. Though easily cured with antibiotics, endocarditis can be life threatening if not treated. Those at greatest risk of developing endocarditis include individuals with congenital heart defects, valve damage due to rheumatic fever, or other valve problems. Also at risk are IV drug users who share contaminated needles.

Heart Failure

The final stage of almost all types of heart disease is heart failure, also known as congestive heart failure. When this occurs, the heart muscle has been weakened to the point where it is unable to pump enough blood to the body.

During the early stages of heart failure, the heart may actually enlarge as it tries to contract more forcefully, but over time, this simply makes the heart function even less efficiently. This causes the kidneys to conserve water in an attempt to increase blood volume, stimulating the heart to pump still harder. Excess fluid eventually seeps from tiny blood vessels into nearby tissue. Fluid can also collect in the lungs (making breathing extremely difficult) and in the ankles, legs, and abdomen. In the final stages of heart failure, physical activity is dramatically reduced to the point where the patient must be bedridden.

The most common cause of congestive heart failure is coronary heart disease. However, heart failure can result from any ailment that damages the heart muscle. People who have repeated heart attacks are extremely susceptible because the attacks kill heart tissue, which in turn makes it increasingly difficult for the heart to pump efficiently.

Heart failure isn't always fatal. Many times it can be reversed or effectively treated for years with the right medication. Digitalis is often prescribed to help the heart pump more effectively, and beta blockers may be used to decrease the heart's workload. In addition, vasodilators may be used to relax the arteries and veins so that blood flows through them more easily, and diuretics may be prescribed to stimulate the kidneys to eliminate excess fluid.

All of these techniques have proved extremely useful. An estimated 4.5 million Americans with heart failure are alive today because of them.

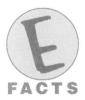

FACTS

It's never too late to give up smoking, report researchers in the *British Medical Journal*. Quitting the tobacco habit even late in life eliminates most of the lung cancer risk, and the risk is decreased more than 90 percent for those who quit before they turn thirty-five.

The Many Facets of Heart Disease

Heart disease is more of an umbrella term than a single diagnosis. In fact, most medical texts discuss more than 100 abnormal conditions of the heart and blood vessels. Here are the ones you're most likely to hear your doctor mention during a checkup:

- *Angina pectoris*—chest pain resulting from a lack of oxygen to the heart, most often due to an insufficient blood supply during times of physical or emotional stress
- *Arrhythmias*—abnormal rhythms or rates of heartbeat
- *Congestive heart failure*—the inability of the heart to maintain its normal pace.
- *Heart valve disease*—a disease that occurs when one or more of the four valves in the heart become defective and disrupt normal blood flow
- *Cardiomyopathy*—abnormal or unusually decreased function of the heart

Arthritis

According to the National Arthritis Foundation, arthritis is one of the most common complaints of old age. It comes in more than 100 different types, afflicts an estimated 40 million Americans, and is the number one cause of physical disability.

Arthritis knows no boundaries. It affects both men and women equally and does not discriminate between race, background, or socioeconomic level. Though most arthritis victims are adults (the vast majority being seniors), arthritis-related conditions also affect nearly 300,000 children in the United States.

Arthritis, in its many forms, most commonly afflicts the joints. But to understand how arthritis causes damage, it's necessary to understand joint physiology. Joints are made of cartilage surrounded by a strong casing known as the joint capsule. The joint capsule is lined with a special membrane that secretes a lubricating liquid known as synovial fluid. Depending on its type, arthritis causes pain, swelling, and stiffness in the joints by affecting the protective cushion where the two bones meet.

Osteoarthritis

The most common type of arthritis is osteoarthritis, also known as degenerative joint disease. This condition afflicts nearly 20 million Americans and is most common in men and women over age fifty-five. It results when the cartilage cushion in the joints breaks down, causing the bones to rub together. Common symptoms of osteoarthritis include pain, stiffness, and sometimes the formation of bone spurs. Though osteoarthritis can affect any joint in the body, it is most commonly found in the hands, feet, spine, hips, and knees.

Osteoarthritis usually results from age-related wear and tear on the joints, though it can often be worsened by injury, repeated joint stress, and obesity. (Excessive weight places additional pressure on weight-bearing joints such as the hips and knees.) A growing body of research suggests that osteoarthritis may also be at least partly hereditary and may be due to genetic abnormalities in the cells that make cartilage.

Inflammatory Arthritis

Inflammatory types of arthritis are also common. Unlike osteoarthritis, which is caused by a degeneration of joint tissue, inflammatory types of arthritis cause joint stiffness and pain by stimulating an inflammation and swelling of the synovial membrane. The inflamed tissue releases special chemicals that increase blood flow to the affected joint, causing it to look red and feel warm to the touch. The best-known type of inflammatory arthritis is rheumatoid arthritis.

Unfortunately, many victims of inflammatory arthritis make the condition worse by favoring the affected joints and holding them in a fixed position to reduce the pain. This can cause the muscles surrounding the joints to weaken and the tendons, which attach muscles to bone or to other muscles, to tighten, resulting in a gradual loss of mobility.

Many types of inflammatory arthritis are the result of an autoimmune reaction, which means the body's disease-fighting cells attack the synovium in the joints. Doctors still aren't sure exactly how this process occurs, though some believe genetics may play a role. However, although some genes are known to predispose people to certain forms of inflammatory arthritis, these genes are not the only factor. Researchers believe other still-unidentified genes may be involved, as well as external triggers such as viruses or environmental agents.

Rheumatoid Arthritis

As noted, rheumatoid arthritis is the most common form of autoimmune-induced arthritis. Extremely painful and frequently disabling, rheumatoid arthritis affects more than 2 million Americans, most of them between the ages of twenty and forty. Inexplicably, it is three times more likely to strike women than men.

Rheumatoid arthritis usually occurs in the same joints on both sides of the body, such as the hands, wrists, shoulders, or knees. The inflammation that results from the immune system's attack on the synovial tissue can lead to extensive joint damage and impede mobility. In extreme cases, the bone itself erodes due to action from the immune cells, causing joints to dislocate and, in turn, to freeze in one position.

Rheumatoid arthritis can also afflict children. In fact, an estimated 71,000 children in the United States are affected by juvenile rheumatoid arthritis, the most common symptoms being joint pain, swelling, and stiffness. Mild cases of the disorder may disappear after a few years, though severe cases can last a lifetime.

There are three specific forms of juvenile rheumatoid arthritis. Systemic JRA, also known as Still's disease, accounts for up to 20 percent of all cases. This form of the disease usually starts as a high fever and rash, followed a few months later by increasing joint pain and swelling. Still's disease can also affect a child's internal organs, including the heart and lungs. Most of these side conditions disappear after a few months, though the arthritis itself may linger into adulthood.

Additional Arthritis Autoimmune Disorders

Rheumatoid arthritis isn't the only arthritis-related autoimmune disorder to afflict adults; also relatively common is lupus erythematosus, or simply lupus. Symptoms of this painful condition include fever, rash, and swelling of the joints. Complications of the disorder can be serious and include inflammation of the heart lining, lungs, kidneys, brain, and bone marrow. Nearly a quarter of a million Americans are afflicted with lupus. Women are five times more likely to develop the disease, which most often strikes younger women between the ages of fifteen and forty.

Even more common is ankylosing spondylitis, which is caused by chronic inflammation of the spine. This bizarre condition usually begins with pain and stiffness in the sacroiliac joint, located between the lower bones in the spinal column. As the disease worsens, joint inflammation around the bones of the spinal column can cause these bones to fuse. Ankylosing spondylitis can also afflict the shoulder, hip, and knee joints.

More than 400,000 Americans are affected by ankylosing spondylitis. The disorder usually develops before age forty and is three times more common in men than women. Research suggests a genetic link to increased risk of the disease; 90 percent of all people with AS carry a specific gene known as the HLA-B27 gene. But because not everyone with the gene develops AS, researchers believe an infectious or environmental trigger may also play a role.

Gout

This type of inflammatory arthritis is different from rheumatoid arthritis and lupus in that it results from deposits of sodium urate crystals in the joints rather than from an autoimmune response. (The crystals result from excess uric acid circulating in the blood.) Unlike other forms of arthritis, which tend to afflict numerous joints, gout usually strikes only one, the most common being a joint in the big toe. Gout is painful and, if left untreated, can become a chronic condition.

An estimated 2 million Americans suffer from gout, which used to be known as a wealthy person's disease because it was thought to result from an extravagant diet. The disease most often afflicts males between the ages of forty and fifty, and up to 20 percent of those afflicted have a family history of the disease. Risk factors include excessive alcohol consumption, obesity, and hypertension.

Lyme Disease

This is one of the best known forms of infectious arthritis and results from a bacterial infection transmitted by the bite of the deer tick. As the infection spreads through the body, it can cause vomiting, fever, neck stiffness, and headaches. If treatment is not received promptly, chronic joint inflammation can result. In most cases, a regimen of antibiotics is all that's necessary to eliminate the infection.

Reiter's Syndrome

This condition is usually a complication of infection of the bowels, urinary tract, or genitals. It comes in two forms. The first is typically related to a sexually transmitted infection such as chlamydia and is the most common cause of arthritis in young men. The second form usually occurs as a result of an intestinal bacteria infection and is more common among the elderly.

The symptoms of Reiter's syndrome include pain and swelling in the joints and tendons and inflammation of the eyes. Some patients experience only one bout of the disorder; in others it becomes chronic. Interestingly, most people who develop Reiter's syndrome carry the HLA-B27 gene, which is also extremely common among those afflicted with ankylosing spondylitis. Like AS, the gene does not appear to cause the disease but predisposes people to an infectious trigger.

Diagnosing and Treating Arthritis

Arthritis in its many forms is usually diagnosed and treated by specialists known as rheumatologists. These doctors use a wide variety of techniques to accurately diagnose arthritis and determine the most appropriate course of treatment. Diagnosis usually begins with a complete physical examination, which includes discussion of the patient's symptoms, medical history, and family history. An examination is also conducted to determine the pattern of joints affected; this information is often extremely helpful in pinpointing the type of arthritis the patient may have.

Inflammatory arthritis is most often diagnosed through the use of laboratory tests, including a blood test that measures how quickly red blood cells cling together and fall to the bottom of a test tube. If the cells sink quickly, inflammation is usually present in the body. Doctors also test a patient's blood or synovial fluid for the presence of specific antibodies, which are activated in the body by infections. Rheumatoid factor antibodies indicate a rheumatoid arthritis; antinuclear antibodies indicate lupus. Sometimes rheumatologists also test for specific genes, such as the HLA-B27 gene, which is common to ankylosing spondylitis.

While certain types of infectious arthritis can be cured with antibiotics, there is no cure for most other forms of the disease. The primary goal of most treatment regimens is a reduction in pain and swelling, the maintenance of mobility, and an improved quality of life. The most common tools used in achieving these goals are pain-relieving and anti-inflammatory drugs, and regular exercise. One of the best forms of exercise for people with arthritis, say rheumatologists, is swimming, which works the muscles with a minimum of joint strain.

The most common medications prescribed for the treatment of arthritis pain and swelling include nonsteroidal anti-inflammatory agents such as aspirin, naproxen, and ibuprofen. For severe inflammation, glucocorticoids may be prescribed. And in extreme cases of rheumatoid arthritis, disease modifying antirheumatic drugs may be required to slow the progress of the disease and prevent a debilitating breakdown of the joints. These drugs include hydroxychloroquine, sulfaslazine, and methotrexate.

Osteoporosis

Osteoporosis is a condition characterized by a gradual decrease in bone mass, resulting in bones that are more porous and easier to break than healthy bones. All bones can be affected by osteoporosis, though fractures of the wrist, spine, and hip are most common. White females are the most susceptible to osteoporosis, particularly those who are postmenopausal, but the condition can also affect older men. Additional risk factors include low calcium intake, lack of exercise, smoking, low body weight, poor nutrition, the use of certain drugs such as corticosteroids, as well as a family history of osteoporosis.

Osteoporosis is so common among the elderly that most people consider it a normal and acceptable part of the aging process rather than a separate—and treatable—disease. The most common form of the disorder is known as primary osteoporosis; it includes postmenopausal, or estrogen-deficient, osteoporosis. This is most frequently seen in women whose ovaries have stopped producing estrogen as a result of menopause.

Other forms of the disorder include age-related osteoporosis, which generally affects men and women over the age of seventy, and idiopathic osteoporosis, a rare condition of unknown cause that strikes premenopausal women and men who are middle-aged or younger. Secondary osteoporosis is usually caused by bone atrophy as a result of paralysis or other conditions. Astronauts often experience secondary osteoporosis as a result of spending extended periods in weightlessness.

In most people, progressive bone loss begins around age twenty but becomes symptomatic around age forty-five in women and fifty-five in men. The condition occurs four times more frequently in women than in men, and more frequently in whites and those of Northern European descent than in blacks.

Causes of Osteoporosis

The cause of osteoporosis remains a mystery, though researchers do know that it is strongly related to low calcium levels and reduced estrogen production in women. In addition, researchers have recently discovered a gene that determines the type of vitamin D receptor a person inherits. One form of the VDR gene produces a receptor that stores calcium more efficiently than the other. People who inherit two copies of the more efficient VDR gene develop thicker, more dense bones. Those who inherit two copies of the less efficient gene tend to have somewhat weaker bones.

Symptoms of Osteoporosis

The most common symptom of osteoporosis is an increase in bone fractures, particularly in the spine, hip, and extremities. (Women over forty-five experience more than 1 million hip fractures each year. Statistically, nearly 40 percent of all white women will have experienced a fractured hip by the time they reach their eightieth birthday.) Older women may also develop a curvature of the spine known colloquially as "dowager's hump," and a reduction in height of up to two inches.

Diagnosing and Treating Osteoporosis

Osteoporosis is usually diagnosed through a thorough medical history and the elimination of all other possible diseases or secondary causes, such as hyperparathyroidism, Cushing's disease, malnutrition, or alcoholism. A bone density test can also confirm the diagnosis. (All women should have a baseline bone density test performed by the time they are forty-five years old.)

Osteoporosis, like most disorders, is easier to prevent than it is to treat. Women (but also men) should consume plenty of calcium throughout their lives, either through a calcium-rich diet or supplements. And this shouldn't stop once a woman enters menopause; an RDA of 1,000 milligrams helps keep bones strong when estrogen levels decrease. Regular weight-bearing exercise, such as walking or swimming, can also help slow bone loss. In addition, women are encouraged to maintain a healthy weight; those who are extremely thin as a result of athletics or dance are more prone to osteoporosis later in life.

Some postmenopausal women opt for synthetic estrogen or progestin therapy to help prevent the effects of osteoporosis. A new synthetic estrogen called raloxifene was approved in 1997 for the treatment of osteoporosis; it increases bone density with fewer side effects than previous types of synthetic estrogen. Nonhormonal treatments include drugs such as calcitonin and alendronate sodium.

Prevention and Aging Diseases

The first step toward adding more years to your life and more life to your years—the goal of all anti-aging research—is to do what you can to prevent or slow the many diseases that occur with age. Not surprisingly, almost all of the disorders we've discussed so far have a lifestyle or environmental component to their development. If you improve your lifestyle and/or your environment, you'll be well on your way to reducing your risk of serious illness.

Heart disease, for example, is often the result of a lifetime of rich, fatty foods, too little exercise, and, typically, years of smoking. If this sounds like you, don't worry; it's never too late to start living more healthfully. The human body is an amazingly resilient machine, and even years of abuse can be corrected with some simple changes in lifestyle. You can reduce your cholesterol level by eating less meat and more fruits, vegetables, grains, and legumes, for instance; doing so will lay the groundwork for keeping your heart healthy and strong for many, many years to come.

The risk of stroke is decreased by controlling high blood pressure. Other risk factors include a diet too high in cholesterol, smoking, and a lack of exercise. If you start eating right, working out more, and avoiding tobacco, you'll be doing both your heart and your brain a favor. They'll repay your efforts with decades more of faithful service.

Many types of cancer, as noted earlier, have a strong nutritional and environmental component. Potentially dangerous foods include those high in fat and low in fiber, grilled or charred meats, and alcohol. (While some studies suggest that moderate alcohol consumption has some beneficial effects, most studies have found a higher rate of cancer among those who drink.) Environmental factors include tobacco use (or breathing secondhand smoke) and exposure to pesticides and other harmful chemicals, which occurs in many occupations.

To hedge your bet against cancer, pack your diet with known cancer-fighting foods such as broccoli, cauliflower, brussels sprouts, tomatoes and tomato products, carrots, citrus fruit, garlic, and onions. The addition of high-fiber foods is also a good idea because fiber helps move food through the digestive system. Examples of high-fiber foods include apples, prunes, brown rice, whole wheat bread, beans, and peas. In addition, avoid environmental pollutants whenever possible, and wear protective clothing and face masks when working with pesticides and other dangerous chemicals.

Osteoporosis is best prevented by making sure you consume plenty of bone-strengthening calcium throughout your life. But again, even if you've been negligent, it's never too late to start eating a calcium-rich diet, choosing calcium-fortified foods, and taking calcium supplements. Exercises, especially weight-bearing activities, are also good for maintaining bone strength and density. And finally, don't smoke; it inhibits calcium absorption.

Because of its very nature, osteoarthritis is more difficult to prevent. However, doctors say you can hedge your bet by avoiding bone and joint injuries (trauma is considered a primary risk factor), eating well, and maintaining your ideal weight. And don't worry that exercise will increase your risk of developing arthritis; several clinical studies have concluded that regular physical activity has no bearing on the formation of the disease in older men and women.

Obesity is one of the primary causes of diabetes, so prevention obviously begins with proper diet and weight maintenance. And, again, regular exercise—meaning at least four times a week—can also help keep this potentially deadly disorder at bay. If you find that you have several of the most common symptoms of diabetes, see your doctor immediately for a diagnostic workup. Early detection can make management easier and, in turn, reduce the risk of serious complications.

Living with Chronic Disease

Regardless of how well we take care of ourselves, the chances are pretty good that we'll eventually end up with some sort of chronic medical condition. This doesn't mean that we did anything wrong or that we could have done something better; it's just a natural part of life. However, many chronic diseases can prematurely age us if we let them. The following tips can help you stay young in the face of chronic illness:

- *Understand your disease.* Many people let chronic illness get the better of them simply because they don't understand how the disease affects their body and, thus, what they must do to keep it under control. Don't hesitate to ask your doctor questions and to make him repeat important information in lay terms if he gets too technical.
- *Follow your doctor's advice.* The word *chronic* means "lasting a long time," so a chronic disease is one that may never go away. As a result, it's easy to become complacent and gradually less attentive regarding the management of a chronic condition. The result is diminished health and more rapid aging. Your doctor can tell you what you must do to keep your condition under control; it's your responsibility to follow his advice as closely as possible. The

management of a chronic condition can be time consuming, but your overall health depends on it.

• *Stay abreast of the latest research.* Advances in medical science are being made every day, some of which may eventually help you in the management of your condition. Read the newspaper, listen to the news, and quiz your doctor on a regular basis. Official organizations such as the American Diabetes Association or the Arthritis Foundation can also help you stay informed; check their Web sites regularly.

• *Join a support group.* Many people find the management of a chronic disease overwhelming to the point where they wonder if it's really worth it. A support group can help you stay motivated in the face of medical adversity. It will also provide camaraderie and friendship.

Genes and the Diseases of Aging

What role will mapping the human genome play in alleviating the many ailments commonly associated with aging? Plenty, say researchers. In fact, medical studies have already started on a variety of fronts.

Take osteoporosis, for example. Long believed to be caused by low calcium levels and diminishing levels of estrogen, a recent report in the journal *Science* noted an association between brittle bones and an enzyme known as cathepsin K. This special enzyme is produced by a class of cells known as osteoclasts, which are responsible for the breakdown of bone. Osteoblasts, on the other hand, are cells that build up bone mass. In healthy individuals, osteoblasts and osteoclasts work in harmony to ensure normal bone growth and maintenance. However, when too much cathepsin K is produced, bones become thinner. Researchers are now working on a drug that would keep osteoporosis from developing (or at least worsening) by inhibiting cathepsin K.

Obesity is another age-related condition that could potentially be aided with genetic research. The biggest question is, Why do some people remain slender no matter how much they eat, while others seem to pile on the pounds regardless of how well they manage their diet? One possible answer, say researchers at the University of California-Davis, could be a gene that is a blueprint for a protein known as UCP2.

Laboratory studies have found that animals with high levels of UCP2 in their tissues tend to maintain a normal, healthy weight, while animals with low levels tend to gain weight very easily. A drug that could stimulate the production of UCP2 could be just what the doctor ordered for the millions of Americans who find themselves unexpectedly gaining weight in their later years.

Genetic research may also result in a cure for Type II diabetes, which commonly afflicts people over fifty and is most prevalent in those who are overweight. Medical research recently discovered two genes in a specific strain of Type II diabetes that adversely affect the body's efforts to metabolize blood sugar. If these genes—which also regulate activity in the intestines, kidneys, and pancreas—could be manipulated through some type of gene therapy, this form of diabetes could be made a thing of the past, say doctors.

CHAPTER 7

Take a Look Around

In this chapter, we'll examine in depth the most common environmental issues facing us today, their influence on our health and longevity, and what you must do to eliminate the most serious hazards. This chapter also places a lot of emphasis on health hazards at home and in the workplace, because that is where we spend so much of our time. There are some life factors that we can't control, such as accidents at the hands of others, but regular vigilance can still improve our quality of life and our hopes for the future.

Longevity and Your Environment

Our environment has just as much impact on our health and longevity as does our diet and lifestyle. In fact, it may very well play an even greater role, because very often the conditions of our environment (air quality, exposure to toxic chemicals, overall safety, etc.) are so subtle or seemingly innocuous that we don't even think about them until it's too late to make necessary changes.

When talking about environment, we mean living conditions, work surroundings, and general outdoor climate; it's a fairly broad umbrella term that encompasses everything from the air quality of your office, to pesticide exposure when working in your garden, to how well you have "accident proofed" your home. All of these and a hundred other factors affect our health (often down to the cellular level) every day and can play a dramatic role in how well we age and how long we live.

As noted, many people take their environment for granted. They just assume that the quality of their air is good, that their water is free of contaminants, and that their home and work environments are safe. But a glance at any newspaper suggests just the opposite. Indeed, every aspect of our environment requires constant monitoring to ensure we're living as well and as healthfully as possible.

Environment is just one aspect of our longevity plan, but it's a vitally important one, more so than many others because it also affects our loved ones. Radon exposure via a cracked cellar floor, for example, means a greater risk of cancer not only to us but also to everyone who spends time in that basement. Similarly, a failure to correct potential accident risks in every room of the house puts every occupant in jeopardy. So you see, a safe and controlled environment means a longer life for everyone concerned.

Common Environmental Hazards

The concept that environmental substances can make people sick is not new. In fact, it was first proposed in the fourth century B.C. by the Greek physician Hippocrates, who suggested that illness could result from air contaminated by a variety of wastes, including the decay of dead plants and animals. The ancient Romans also understood this concept, noting the potential for disease from exposure to environmental toxins such as mercury, lead, and even asbestos.

FACTS

A great many organisms in nature have achieved extreme longevity, while to humans it is still only a pipe dream. The oldest known organism on Earth is the bristlecone pine, which lives high in the California and Nevada mountains. One such tree was believed to be almost 4,900 years old when it was cut down in 1964.

The biggest lesson researchers have learned in studying long-lived animals and plants is the importance of a safe environment. Very simply, certain creatures are able to live longer and age more slowly because they don't have to worry about predators or disease.

Today, awareness of the impact our environment can have on us has never been higher. Depending on where we live, we question the quality of the air we breathe, the water we drink, and the food we eat. Is it safe? Could it be safer? And how about our work environment? Is our building "sick"? Are we being exposed to toxic chemicals?

In today's world, it's easy to become paranoid, especially if you regularly read the newspaper or watch the evening news. Every day, it seems, researchers are discovering that something we've long taken for granted as safe is, in fact, harmful to our health. Just how much trouble are we in, anyway?

That's a difficult question to answer. Certain environmental risks are unquestionable; others are open to serious debate. And the issue is clouded further as researchers learn more about the effects certain chemicals and compounds have on the human body and try to ascertain their risk. It's accurate to say that the majority of Americans are relatively safe from the most serious environmental hazards, though constant monitoring is important because the situation can change in a heartbeat. A municipal water source, for example, can be pure one day and contaminated the next, requiring users to either boil their drinking water or buy bottled water until the problem has been corrected. Fortunately, such situations are usually quickly reported by the local press and corrected without delay. But if you don't know about the problem, your risk of exposure to potential health hazards is high.

It's important not to let your fears get the best of you. Scary news story after scary news story can cause even the most rational persons to question virtually everything in their environment. But as long as you remain knowledgeable and aware, you and your family should have nothing to worry about.

Routes of Exposure

Before we look at environmental issues in the home, at work, and outside, it's important that you understand the three basic routes of exposure to environmental agents. They are the skin, gastrointestinal tract, and lungs.

The skin is our first line of defense in protecting the inside of the body from the outside environment. Skin is tough and offers very good protection from most pollutants, but it's not perfect. Harmful agents can enter the bloodstream if the protective layer of waxy liquid on the skin's surface is broken or dissolved. As a result, it's always a good idea to wear sufficient protection when working with potentially dangerous chemicals, such as cleaning products, pesticides, and solvents.

The gastrointestinal tract protects our internal organs from harmful agents that are ingested. Exposure can occur when soluble compounds are consumed, absorbed, and then taken into the cells.

The lungs are considered the most important—and the most vulnerable—route of exposure to environmental toxins. Potentially dangerous airborne agents can be deposited in the lungs and, if soluble, absorbed into the bloodstream. Our lungs are sturdy organs that work hard without a break throughout our lives, but they are very susceptible to certain agents. Smokers are at particular risk because their lungs have already taken a beating.

Water Pollution

Water is essential for human life; without it, we die within days. Water is known as the "universal solvent" because of its amazing ability to pick up other substances after the briefest of exposures. As a result, pure water—that is, water consisting only of H_2O—does not exist in nature. All water has something else in it.

Water's ability to attract other chemicals is vital to our very survival. We depend on it to transport nutrients to cells and carry away cellular wastes, and some minerals found naturally in water, such as calcium, magnesium, and iron, are important to cellular survival. But when the water we drink picks up pollutants, problems occur.

Water pollution has been a public issue and a public worry for decades. In fact, according to one national survey, 70 percent of Americans are worried about the quality of the water they drink.

The Most Dangerous Water Pollutants

Many people believe that they can tell whether the water they drink is safe by its clarity, taste, or odor. However, that's not always true. Sometimes water that is a tad murky or somewhat off tasting (such as sulfur water or well water containing manganese or iron) is perfectly fine to drink, while water that appears crystal clear is actually full of contaminants, such as lead. Unless a pollution problem is very obvious, it usually takes laboratory testing to accurately determine water quality.

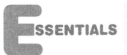

Here are some tips for reducing lead in your drinking water:

- Do not use hot water for cooking or drinking because it tends to dissolve more lead from pipes. Always use cold water, especially when preparing foods for infants and young children.
- Upon awakening, let tap water run for several minutes before drinking. The reason: Lead concentrations are highest when water has sat in pipes for several hours. Flushing the toilet and running the shower for a few minutes can also help drain pipes of standing water.
- Throughout the day, let tap water run for several seconds before drinking.

Under the Safe Drinking Water Act of 1974, the federal government regulates more than sixty contaminants that may appear in municipal water supplies. Let's take a closer look at some of the contaminants that you should be most aware of.

Microorganisms

Before the widespread use of chlorinating and other disinfecting techniques, waterborne microorganisms were a constant health hazard, resulting in such potentially deadly diseases as cholera, dysentery, and typhoid fever. Today, the threat from microorganisms is much less than a century ago, but no water supply is ever 100 percent protected, say environmental experts. The risk of contamination is always a possibility, and you should pay close attention to area news sources for warnings and information. Contamination from microorganisms such as bacteria and viruses is especially likely when municipal water mains are broken or breached during a natural disaster such as a hurricane or flood, though sometimes accidents occur during construction. When contamination is a possibility, users are urged to boil their water before drinking or to use bottled water until the problem can be fixed. Most of the time, such problems are corrected within a day or two.

Most microbial outbreaks occur in surface water sources, but groundwater sources are also at risk. Private wells and municipal underground water supplies can become contaminated with bacteria from leaking septic tanks or animal waste that soaks into the ground. If you get your water from a well and live in farm country, near a landfill, or in an industrial area, you should have your water checked by a laboratory on a regular basis, just to be on the safe side.

Organic Chemicals

A variety of organic chemicals can contaminate a water supply, including pesticides, herbicides, and industrial wastes. Many of them cannot be detected through odor, color, or flavor, but in high concentrations, these chemicals can cause severe illness and even death.

Toone, Tennessee, experienced organic chemical contamination at its worst. Between 1964 and 1973, the Vesicol Chemical Company buried nearly 200,000 drums of pesticide waste material in shallow pits on its farm near Toone. The hazardous chemicals seeped out and contaminated the wells of nearby residents, many of whom developed nausea, breathing problems, severe fatigue, and kidney and liver ailments. One well that supplied drinking water to six families was found to contain levels of carbon tetrachloride that were 2,400 times the maximum allowed by the U.S. Environmental Protection Agency. In 1986, after a prolonged legal battle, a Tennessee court awarded the residents of Toone $5 million in medical and property compensation and $7.5 million in punitive damages.

What happened in Toone is an extreme example of water pollution. However, organic chemicals can also leach into water supplies in very small amounts, sometimes measured in parts per billion. It is generally assumed that consumption of these chemicals in such small quantities poses little risk to our health, though there is very little research into the effects of such consumption over extended periods. As a result, some researchers warn of a possible lifetime increase in risk of cancer and other disorders.

Organic contamination can come from a number of possible sources. Some contamination occurs naturally, the result of animal and vegetable decay or the deposit of soil into the water. Not surprisingly, natural contamination occurs much more frequently in surface water than in groundwater sources, because surface supplies are often open and unprotected.

FACTS

By the time most of us reach our sixtieth birthday, our eyes have been exposed to the amount of light energy produced by a nuclear blast.

Other organics, such as pesticides, herbicides, and industrial waste, are man made. They often find their way into surface water sources by seeping through waste sites or via intentional (and illegal) dumping. Farms and ranches can be big sources of organic contamination if care is not taken with waste disposal.

Some of the most worrisome and controversial organic water pollutants are chlorination by-products known as trihalomethanes (THMs), which result when chlorine—one of the most common water disinfectants—reacts with naturally occurring organic matter such as dead plants. The most dangerous THM is chloroform, which is believed to cause cancer in humans.

Another organic water pollutant of concern is the family of chlorinated hydrocarbons, which are widely used as industrial solvents. These chemicals are often found in industrial effluents and are frequently discharged into rivers and lakes, where they can contaminate drinking supplies by soaking through the soil into groundwater. Individuals most at risk of chlorinated hydrocarbon contamination live near toxic waste sites, landfills, and even military bases.

The health risk from exposure to chlorinated hydrocarbons is substantial. In high doses, the chemicals can damage the nervous system, liver, and kidneys, and there is some evidence that they also can cause cancer.

Aromatic hydrocarbons, which include toluene, xylene, and benzene, are another family of organic chemicals that can pose a danger if they find their way into our drinking water. Benzene is a known human carcinogen, and all of the chemicals in this group can cause problems with fetal development when ingested in high amounts.

Sources of aromatic hydrocarbons include leaky gasoline storage tanks, industrial runoff, and improper disposal of cleaning fluids by home owners. Once they soak into the ground, it's easy for these chemicals to find their way into surface water and groundwater drinking supplies.

Heavy Metals

When referring to heavy metal in this context, we're not talking about big hair and ear-splitting rock music. Environmentally speaking, heavy metals are elements, such as lead, mercury, and cadmium, that can be quite bad for our health—should they be found in high concentrations in our drinking water.

Heavy metals can leach into water supplies from a variety of different sources. The most common is aging landfills, which can dump heavy metals into nearby groundwater. However, heavy metals can also find their way into municipal water supplies when dumped into sewers by metal-finishing companies, or into our home tap water via corroded pipes. Of the latter, lead, cadmium, and copper are the most frequently detected.

Ingesting even small amounts of heavy metals can be bad for our health. In addition to interfering with a variety of body processes, heavy metals can damage the brain, nervous system, and kidneys, and cause male infertility. Fetuses and infants are particularly sensitive to the effects of heavy metals, particularly lead.

Indeed, lead poses one of the greatest health threats when it comes to our water. In high doses, this metal, which once was commonly used in household plumbing, can cause severe brain damage and even death; in low doses, it can cause nerve system damage in still-developing fetuses, infants, and children. The most common effects include learning disabilities and hyperactive behavior.

Modern construction has eliminated the risk of lead poisoning in new houses (both in plumbing and lead-based paint), though the danger may still exist in older structures that have not had their plumbing replaced. Those most at risk are individuals living in homes constructed between 1910 and 1940, when lead service pipes were commonly used. However, somewhat newer houses may also have lead pipes, particularly in colder regions where lead pipes were preferred because of their resistance to cracks during freezing weather. Also risky are homes with plumbing consisting of copper pipes connected by lead-based solder (which was banned by federal law in 1986) and older chrome-plated bathroom fixtures, which are made of brass consisting of 3 to 8 percent lead.

Radon

This naturally occurring radioactive gas is formed when uranium decays, and it poses a very serious health threat, especially when it gets into our drinking water. In fact, many environmental experts believe waterborne radon may be responsible for more cancer deaths than all other drinking-water contaminants combined.

According to the Environmental Protection Agency, inhaled indoor radon results in between 5,000 and 20,000 lung cancer deaths annually.

Most of these deaths are the result of radon gas rising up from the ground and accumulating in homes through cracks in basements and foundations. However, a small percentage—perhaps up to 1,800 deaths per year—are believed to be caused by radon in household water. In this case, however, the health hazard is not from the consumption of contaminated water but from radon dissolved in the water escaping into the indoor air when water is sprayed in showers and washing machines. According to EPA estimates, up to 8 million Americans may have dangerously high levels of radon in their household water, with the risk being limited to people who use groundwater.

Nitrates

Drinking water typically provides around 1 percent of a person's daily intake of nitrates, with the rest coming from vegetables. But in some areas of the country, water supplies from private wells in farming areas may contain dangerously high levels of these chemicals, which usually result from the use of chemical fertilizers and manure. However, water from leaking septic tanks can also contaminate groundwater with nitrates.

Those most at risk of nitrate exposure are infants younger than six months old. Consuming formula made with water contaminated with nitrates can result in a dangerous condition known as methemoglobinemia, in which the blood has difficulty transporting oxygen. Symptoms include shortness of breath and weakness.

While water contamination from other sources seems to be improving in most parts of the country, the EPA warns that nitrate pollution seems to be getting worse, particularly in rural areas. As a result, rural well users with new babies are encouraged to have their water checked periodically for nitrates and other contaminants.

Is Your Water Safe?

As noted earlier, color, flavor, and odor are not accurate tests of your water's purity. If you have the slightest suspicion that your water may be contaminated, it should be tested in a laboratory.

If you use a municipal water supply that services more than 500 people, the utilities department is required by federal law to test its water regularly and make the findings of those tests available to the public free of charge. So the first thing you should do if you have any questions regarding your drinking water is contact your local water company and ask for the last complete analysis.

It's important to note that this analysis will tell you the quality of the water when it left the treatment plant—not necessarily as it pours out of your household tap. As a result, your household water may contain higher levels of lead, for example, than the analysis reports because lead has leached into your water through municipal or household pipes on its way from the treatment plant to your faucet. If you don't trust the quality of your water, it might be a good idea to have it tested by a private lab. Such an analysis can be tailored for a wide spectrum of possible pollutants, or just one or two.

People who get their water from a private well are at greater risk of poor water quality than those who are served by a treated municipal water supply. If you fear your water is less than pure, contact your local public health department and ask about groundwater contamination in your area. Environmental experts suggest that well users have their water tested annually for bacteria, radon, and inorganic chemicals. If you live within a mile of a landfill, gas station, military base, or chemical plant, make sure you also have your water tested for organic chemicals. And those living in rural areas should be wary of nitrate, pesticide, and herbicide contamination.

For the most accurate results, have your water tested by an independent, state-certified testing laboratory. If there is no testing laboratory within your area, contact your local health department for recommendations regarding mail-order testing laboratories. Foremost, stay away from companies that sell water-treatment equipment. Many such companies offer free water testing, but it's certain that they won't be objective; the test is just a way of getting you to buy a water treatment kit.

If the analysis shows a high concentration of a particular contaminant, get a second opinion from another laboratory before taking corrective measures. Most laboratory results are accurate, but there is always the possibility of a false reading, and you don't want to waste money on a filtration system or other steps you don't really need.

Air Pollution

Air pollution isn't something that's limited to big cities or industrial regions; it can also afflict small towns and rural communities. Nor is air pollution strictly an "outdoor event." Some of the worst air pollution, from a health and longevity perspective, can be found in our homes and places of work.

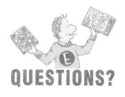

QUESTIONS?

Do you know what lies beneath the surface of your skin?
Skin is comprised of three layers: the epidermis, the dermis, and the subcutaneous tissue. The epidermis, which is the outermost layer, is as thick as a piece of paper and is comprised of layers of specialized skin cells called keratinocytes. Directly under the epidermis is the dermis, which contains the blood vessels that feed both the skin and the collagen and elastin, special proteins that give the skin its elasticity. The subcutaneous tissue is the bottom layer of the skin. Its main function is to provide insulation and protection for the skin, bones, and organs.

It used to be that towns viewed air pollution as the price of growth and success. Smoke-spewing factories meant jobs, and jobs meant prosperity. So what if you had a nagging, hacking cough? At least everyone was working.

Of course, the situation is quite different today. Air pollution is viewed as a major health hazard and something not to be tolerated. The Environmental Protection Agency and other government bodies have come down hard on industries previously known as major polluters in an attempt to cleanse public air and ensure the safety and health of all Americans. Particularly effective was the Clean Air Act of 1970 and its amendments, which forced industries to reduce their use of soft coal and heavy oil and required factories to place special filters on smoke stacks to reduce the amount of airborne pollutants they spilled into the air.

But despite these efforts, air pollution in various forms continues in this and other countries and still poses a variety of health risks to various populations—health risks that can result in premature aging as well as reduced longevity. Indeed, air pollution is still considered one of the world's most important environmental issues, and rightly so.

How Air Pollution Affects Our Health

Anyone who has lived in an area where smog alerts are common knows the symptoms of breathing dirty air; they include an irritated throat, respiratory problems, watery eyes, and so forth. Known as "transient ailments," these symptoms may also include skin rashes, headaches, nausea, and dizziness. However, chronic exposure to outdoor air pollution, such as that experienced by people living in overcrowded urban areas or factory towns, can also lead to a variety of dangerous chronic health conditions such as emphysema, bronchitis, asthma, and even cancer.

Outdoor air pollution adversely affects the health of everyone who breathes it, though some sensitive populations may feel it worse than others. Those most at risk of aggravated health problems from moderate to extreme air pollution include the elderly (specifically those over sixty-five years of age), the very young (infants and toddlers), and individuals with chronic health conditions such as respiratory ailments and heart disease. These individuals should pay close attention to air quality reports in their area and stay indoors with the air conditioner running when the pollution index is high.

Air Pollution Sources

Air pollution comes from a wide variety of sources. Interestingly, nature itself is a contributor; volcanoes and forest fires pour a huge amount of ash, particles, and dangerous gases into the atmosphere all over the world. But in the big picture, nature has nothing on man when it comes to polluting the air. It's no exaggeration to say we're our own worst enemy.

The combustion of fossil fuels is the biggest culprit, say environmental researchers. Cars pour a huge amount of pollution into the atmosphere every day, particularly in countries where lead fuel is still in use. Power plants and industrial factories also release a lot of gases and particles, despite federal clean-air efforts. Even if a factory is able to reduce pollution emission by 90 percent, which is good, some pollution still makes it into the air we breathe.

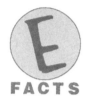

FACTS

The elimination of dead skin cells is a never-ending process. Over the course of our lives, we shed about 40 pounds of skin.

According to ongoing air quality analysis, the worst primary air pollutants are carbon oxides such as the carbon monoxide released by cars, trucks, and buses; sulfur oxides; nitrogen oxides; volatile organic compounds such as hydrocarbons, carbon tetrachloride, and chlorofluorocarbons; and particulate matter such as ash.

Secondary pollutants are formed when primary pollutants react with various chemicals in the atmosphere. The most troublesome include ozone, photochemical oxidants, and particulates in either solid or gas form, such as sulfuric acid and nitric acid. It's these compounds that scientists refer to when discussing "acid rain," a form of air pollution known to devastate forest areas.

Despite government efforts to reduce air emissions, the amount of dangerous substances released into the atmosphere by homes, cars, factories, and power plants every year is staggering. According to the Environmental Protection Agency, billions of pounds (yep, that's billions) of the nearly 15,000 airborne chemicals believed to affect human health are released into the air we breathe every year.

Indoor Air Pollution

If you think that staying home all day will protect you from air pollution, you're wrong. Because most homes are sealed tight due to the use of air conditioners, many potentially harmful substances cannot escape into the atmosphere, so instead they build up inside our homes until, very often, they reach levels higher than air pollutants outdoors!

Some indoor air pollutants, such as radon gas or airborne mold, occur naturally; others, such as tobacco smoke, are the result of our lifestyle. And as strange as it may sound, many different indoor pollutants are emitted by our material possessions, such as formaldehyde fumes from carpeting and processed wood, and carbon monoxide from poorly vented gas stoves and heating units. There's no way to escape it; modern living often means polluted air. Let's take a look at some of the more prevalent forms of indoor pollution.

Asbestos

The use of asbestos as a building material was banned in 1974, but so much of the stuff was used as fireproofing in construction prior to the ban that it is still considered a serious indoor air pollutant—and rightly so. Asbestos fibers are well known for their ability to cause lung cancer and other serious respiratory problems, including asbestosis and bronchogenic carcinoma.

Asbestos poses no hazard as long as it remains intact. However, should it be torn apart during construction or demolition, or simply start to break down from age, fibers can be released into the air and eventually inhaled.

If your house was constructed before the 1974 asbestos construction ban, there is a considerable chance that it contains asbestos in some form. The most common uses for the material included ceiling, roof, and shingle insulation; grout and other paint-patching substances; and steam-pipe insulation, which was made predominantly from asbestos. In addition, many older ovens, dishwashers, and other appliances were wrapped in asbestos insulation.

If you suspect that your house contains asbestos, do not try to remove it yourself! It should be removed ONLY by qualified professionals wearing special protective garments and breathing apparatus. Attempting to rip out asbestos insulation yourself can pour huge amounts of the dangerous fibers into the air, dramatically increasing the risk of cancer not only for yourself but also for everyone else in the vicinity.

Formaldehyde

Anyone who had to dissect a frog in high school biology knows the distinctive stench of formaldehyde, which is commonly used as a biological preservative. Unfortunately, formaldehyde is also used in the manufacture of a wide number of household products, including plywood, particle board, paneling, counter tops, flooring, and carpeting. These products often exude formaldehyde in a process known as "outgassing," resulting in chronic respiratory problems in millions of Americans.

There is also some evidence that exposure to formaldehyde may increase cancer risk. Epidemiologic evidence is considered inconclusive, but several studies offer food for thought. For example, in one study of morticians and pathologists, who are occupationally exposed to formaldehyde in embalming fluid, there appeared to be a higher rate of brain cancer and leukemia. A separate study of British chemical workers exposed to formaldehyde also found a higher than normal incidence of death due to lung cancer.

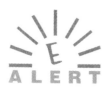

ALERT

The air pollution in Mexico City is some of the worst in the world, due to the city's geography, weather conditions, numerous cars, and unchecked industry. In fact, the lead content in Mexico City's air pollution is so high that female diplomats are encouraged to return to their native countries should they become pregnant to ensure the safety of their unborn babies.

Almost anyone who buys consumer products can expect some exposure to formaldehyde, though those living in newly built tract homes, condominiums, townhouses, and mobile homes risk greater exposure because they tend to use more products known to contain the chemical. In one telling study, a random survey of 470 mobile homes in California found that nearly a third had higher than expected levels, and the Environmental Protection Agency speculates that levels may be high in as many as half of the nation's mobile homes.

If you suffer from unexplained respiratory problems, headaches, or other mysterious symptoms, you could be the victim of formaldehyde exposure. To reduce your risk, air out items known to contain high levels of the chemical, such as new furniture and carpeting, before bringing it into your home.

Radon

We discussed waterborne radon gas earlier, but it poses an equally important hazard when levels build up in our household air. Warnings about the risks radon poses have been touted in the press for years, yet many people fail to really consider how serious a problem it can be and, thus, may be placing their family's health in jeopardy. If this sounds like you, here's a wake-up call: Indoor exposure to radon gas and chemicals in the workplace are considered by the Environmental Protection Agency to be the two primary common causes of cancer.

Radon gas is released into the soil by the decay of uranium-238. It makes its way into houses through cracks in the foundation, basement, and floors. The gas itself also decays, forming tiny particles that attach to dust floating in the air. When these contaminated dust particles are inhaled, they can lodge in the lungs, damaging cells and resulting in cancer.

Radon gas is measured in picocuries per liter of air, and the Environmental Protection Agency has established 4 picocuries per liter of air as the maximum acceptable level within a home. An exposure level of just 15 picocuries per liter of air increases cancer risk to that of a one-pack-a-day smoker. Worse, cancer risk is intensified if there are smokers in the house, because radon acts synergistically with cigarette smoke.

Tobacco Smoke

According to government studies, tobacco smoke is the single largest source of indoor air pollution. Secondhand smoke has been linked to thousands of lung cancer deaths annually, as well as to higher incidences of respiratory problems and chronic ear infections in children. Food for thought: Children whose parents smoke in the house also face an increased risk of lung cancer and other serious disorders.

The dangers of smoking—and of inhaling secondhand smoke—become evident when you understand the number and type of toxic substances released when tobacco is burned. One of the most worrisome is benzene, an extremely harmful substance that is believed to be responsible for many cases of leukemia. The levels of benzene can be extremely high in a closed home with many smokers, and anyone breathing such polluted air faces serious health risks over time.

Improving Air Quality in Your Home

It's never too late to improve the air quality in your home. After all, that's where you and your family spend the majority of your time. You eat at home, sleep at home, and spend your leisure hours at home. Why not make it as environmentally safe, from an air quality perspective, as you can? In so doing, you'll improve your health and add active years to your life.

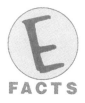

FACTS

The word *smog* was coined decades ago to describe the thick, foggy mixture of pollutants created by the industrial burning of soft coal and heavy oil. In the United States, the word *smog* usually refers to photochemical air pollution formed when certain pollutants emitted directly into the atmosphere react to sunlight to form a mixture containing a number of other different chemical compounds. The most important component of smog in the United States today is ozone. When your local weather person mentions a "smog alert" in your area, he or she is referring to a high ozone concentration. Sensitive individuals should take heed.

Your first step, of course, should be to identify all potential sources of indoor air pollution, then take the necessary steps to eliminate them. Walk from room to room and note all possible problems, such as badly vented heaters, appliances in poor repair, and a lack of early warning systems such as carbon monoxide and radon detectors.

In addition, make sure you review all lifestyle issues that could adversely affect the air quality in your home, such as tobacco use, the frequent use of chemical cleaning agents and solvents, and even chemicals used in hobbies, such as industrial glue or paint. Every time you use such items without taking proper precautions, such as opening windows for ventilation and using a respirator, you pollute the air you breathe and endanger your health. Following are some additional tips to keep the air in your home as clean as possible:

- Avoid all tobacco use indoors. If you simply can't quit, at least take your habit outdoors. And make sure family and friends don't smoke indoors either.
- Make sure your home is well ventilated. Open all the windows whenever possible and consider exhaust fans or air-to-air heat-exchanging devices that draw fresh air in through one duct and expel it through another. In addition, make sure stoves and heaters all vent outdoors. Keeping your house constantly closed tight not only prevents harmful pollutants from dissipating but also promotes sick building syndrome.
- Keep all gas appliances in good working order and have your furnace checked regularly by a qualified professional.
- Have your home checked at least once for radon, especially if you have a basement. If levels are high, take the necessary steps to improve ventilation.
- If your house is somewhat older, bring in a specialist to determine if your insulation is made of asbestos. If the answer is yes, hire a qualified professional to remove it.
- Substitute water-based products for hydrocarbon-based cleaners, which emit dangerous fumes.
- Use environmentally safe products, such as cleaners made from natural ingredients rather than caustic chemicals.
- If you do use products that emit fumes, make sure cans and bottles are tightly closed before you put them away.

- Always use paints and other hazardous chemicals in well-ventilated areas—preferably outdoors.
- When buying home furnishings, select fabrics that do not have a high pile, which can collect dust and other pollutants. And air out any items that may emit formaldehyde fumes before bringing them into your home.
- Try to maintain a humidity level of no more than 50 percent to prevent water from condensing on building materials.
- Ventilate attic and crawlspaces.
- Clean and dry water-damaged rugs and carpets as quickly as possible to prevent the growth of mold and bacteria.

Indoor air pollution is a serious issue that requires constant monitoring and maintenance. As noted, pollutants are often invisible and odorless, so we may not even know they are there until it's too late. That's why it's wise to give your home a quick but thorough check at least once a month.

Safety-Checking Your Home

Living long and well requires much more than eating with proper nutrition in mind, taking the right life-extending supplements, exercising regularly, and enjoying a healthful lifestyle. It also means not dying by accident at home or at work.

It sounds simple enough; just be careful. Yet thousands of people still die in accidents every year. Our home may be our castle, but in many cases, it's also several rooms full of accidents waiting to happen. The reason? Failure to do a basic safety check and take the necessary precautions.

Our intent isn't to frighten you where you live, but to make you pause and take notice. When was the last time you really did a thorough safety check of your home? If you're like most Americans, you probably never have. Perhaps you've thought about it but just never found the time. Sadly, that's the mentality that costs lives, possibly your own.

Home safety is especially important if you have small children or senior citizens living with you. Children, particularly toddlers, are at high risk for serious accidents because of their naturally inquisitive nature; seniors are at risk because of physical impairment and/or limited faculties.

The good news is that most "accidents in waiting" are easy to correct. Very often it's simply a matter of adding rails to a staircase or placing safety stripping under throw rugs. But these things won't take care of themselves; you have to do it. We'll take you through a room-by-room safety checklist so that you know what to watch for.

Kitchen

- All household products and cleaning supplies should be completely inaccessible to small children. Better still, keep them in a locked cupboard in the basement or garage—anywhere but in the kitchen. Check them regularly and safely dispose of old containers.
- All sharp objects, such as knives and scissors, should be safely stored.
- All appliance cords should be out of reach.
- Pot handles should be turned inward when cooking to prevent little hands from grabbing them and to keep them from being accidentally bumped by people walking by.
- Snacks should be well hidden to prevent adventurous children from climbing on counters to get them.

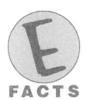

FACTS

The risk of dying from fire is twice as high in homes that do not have functioning fire alarms.

Bathroom

- The medicine chest should be cleaned regularly and outdated medications disposed of properly. In addition, make sure the medicine cabinet is inaccessible to small children.
- Small appliances should be unplugged and out of reach. Never keep small appliances near the bathtub; they can cause electrocution.
- Bathtubs and showers should have safety rails and nonslip decals, especially if used by older people or those with a physical disability.

- A first-aid kit and manual should be readily available in case of emergency.

Bedroom

- Never keep medication on dresser tops or bedside tables where small children can reach it.
- Keep all perfumes and cosmetics out of reach and out of vision.
- Small electrical appliances should be unplugged and out of reach.
- Children's sleeping equipment, including cribs and beds, should be examined regularly to make sure they are properly maintained and free of dangerous defects.

Laundry and Basement

- Detergent and cleaning products should be stored where children cannot reach them.
- Paint, paint remover, solvents, and other dangerous chemicals should be inaccessible.
- All work tools should be unplugged and stored out of reach.
- The furnace area should be clear and free of clutter.
- A first-aid kit and manual should be readily available.

Living Area

- All plants should be safe and nontoxic to humans and animals. If you're unsure whether a plant is poisonous, call a garden store or your local poison control center. If still in doubt, replace it with a plant you know is safe.
- All rugs should be skid proof.
- All staircases should have railings.
- Furniture should be arranged so that children have room to safely play.
- If you have very young children, all furniture with sharp corners should have safety padding (available at most retail and child-specialty stores).
- Venetian blind and drapery cords should be tucked away so that adults won't trip over them and children won't play with them. Warning: These cords can also pose a safety hazard to inquisitive pets.

- Breakable ornaments and knickknacks should be kept out of reach.
- Childproof caps should cover electrical outlets.
- All extension cords should be in good condition. Replace those that are frayed or have cuts in their exterior covering.
- Balcony doors and second floor windows should be locked.

Garage

- All entrances should be securely locked, especially if hazardous chemicals or tools are stored within.
- The garage area should be well lit; stairways leading into it should have handrails and steps should be coated with nonskid paint.
- All power tools and other dangerous machinery should be locked away or stored on a high, sturdy shelf so that inquisitive young children can't reach them. Also, make sure all tools are well secured so that they can't fall and injure someone.
- Paint, varnish, paint thinner, turpentine, and other hazardous chemicals should be stored in childproof containers and locked away.
- Never leave house pets in the garage area, especially if you have laid down mousetraps and other potentially hazardous materials to eliminate vermin. Rat poison is as dangerous to dogs and cats (and young children) as it is to rats.
- Never idle your car in a closed garage; the resulting carbon monoxide can be deadly. If you must warm up your car, make sure the garage door is wide open to allow for ventilation and never let the vehicle idle for more than a minute or two.
- Clean up all spills in the garage area immediately so that they don't pose a hazard to you or others.

Front Yard and Backyard

- Recreational areas should be kept free of dangerous debris such as broken limbs, as well as animal droppings and other hazards.
- Pools—both above and below ground—should be surrounded by a fence with a locked gate. Flotation devices should be readily available.
- All play equipment should be checked and repaired regularly. If an item becomes rusty or broken, throw it away.

- Yards should be free of poisonous plants.
- Sandboxes should be covered to prevent domestic and wild animals from getting into them.

Creating a First-Aid Kit

A first-aid kit should contain the following:

- A selection of adhesive bandages
- A selection of bandage compresses
- Syrup of ipecac to induce vomiting (Syrup of ipecac is recommended for some—but not all—poison emergencies. Never induce vomiting without talking to a doctor first.)
- Sterile eye pads
- A tube of burn ointment
- A tube of antibiotic cream
- An oral antihistamine to diminish an allergic reaction
- A bee sting kit
- Adhesive tape
- A bottle of aspirin and a bottle of acetaminophen (children under twelve should never be given aspirin because of the risk of Reyes's syndrome)
- A roll of adhesive tape
- Bandage scissors
- Tweezers
- A flashlight
- Paper cups
- A blanket
- An eyewash cup
- A card containing the phone numbers of your regional poison control center, the nearest hospital, and your personal physician

Accident Prevention

Are you one of those people who believe that serious accidents are something that happen to the other guy? You're not alone; a great many Americans go about their daily business completely oblivious to the potential accidents they encounter every day at home, work, and elsewhere.

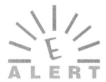

Hobbies are supposed to be a fun way to relax after a hard day at the office, but some hobbies can pose serious environmental hazards if adequate precautions are not taken. The most common hazards facing hobbyists are exposure to toxic chemicals via the skin and inhalation of toxic fumes. Some compounds can make you sick after a single exposure; others require repeated exposures before health problems become evident. Potential health problems range from minor skin rashes or burns to acute respiratory disease, chronic lung disease, and heart, liver, and kidney damage.

According to government statistics, an estimated 150,000 Americans die from injuries every year and more than 60 percent of these deaths are believed to be accidental. Of that number, 80 percent of accidental deaths could have been prevented if simple precautions were taken.

How are Americans dying by accident? The top three killers of American adults aged thirty-five to forty-five are accidental poisoning (primarily drug overdoses), motor vehicle accidents, and firearm accidents, according to the National Center for Health Statistics. Motor vehicle accidents are the third most common cause of death among Americans under age sixty-five, taking more than 45,000 lives and injuring a staggering 500,000 people each year.

The moral: If you want to live to a ripe old age, use common sense to prevent the most common types of lethal accidents. For example, always wear your seat belt when driving or riding in a motor vehicle. The simple fact is that seat belts save lives, which is why most states have enacted strict seat belt laws. But there's also a longevity consideration to seat belt use; serious injuries sustained in the typical motor vehicle accident can accelerate aging by stressing and damaging internal organs and reducing physical activity. If you can't move well, you probably won't exercise regularly. And we already know how lack of exercise can adversely affect the aging process.

Firearm accidents are equally preventable. Misuse of firearms is one of the leading causes of gun accidents, so if you own a gun, take a certification course to learn how to use it properly. Similarly, you should store your gun and ammunition in lockboxes in separate areas of the house and purchase a sturdy gun lock if you have children. Don't fall victim to the assumption that you can safely hide a loaded gun in your house. Children are naturally curious and inquisitive; if a gun is within their reach, they'll find it. Triple check that your gun is unloaded before cleaning it, and NEVER aim a gun—loaded or unloaded—at another person, even in jest. Too many accidental shooting reports contain the phrase "I didn't think it was loaded."

Here are a few more accident prevention tips:

- Always wear a helmet when riding a bicycle or motorcycle. In addition, make sure you wear reflective clothing, even when riding in the daytime.
- Avoid obviously risky household projects, such as climbing up on a steep roof to clean the gutters or chimney. If you can't reach a high area safely from a ladder, hire a professional to do the work for you.
- Follow all of the manufacturer's safety advice when using tools and machinery. Those words of caution are there for a reason.
- Dress properly for all work projects. Always wear protective clothing when using tools and machinery, including goggles when sawing or drilling and ear protectors when machinery is particularly loud. Never think: "I can get away without using protective gear just this once." It only takes one accident to put you in the hospital.
- Never try to "improve" the function of tools or machinery. And if a repair is obviously beyond your skill, let the pros handle it.

Is Your Job Killing You?

When most people hear the phrase "occupational hazards," they immediately think of police officers, firefighters, or circus lion tamers—occupations that by their very nature are dangerous. But even office workers can be exposed to occupational health hazards. Granted, they don't have to worry about crooks with guns, out of control fires, or angry cats, but the risk to their health can be just as great, say environmental health experts.

The idea of occupational hazards is not a new one. As far back as the seventeenth century, physicians were encouraged to ask patients about their profession as part of a standard medical examination, the rationale being that certain jobs could result in very specific health problems. Two centuries later, Dr. Alice Hamilton, the first doctor in the United States to specialize in occupational medicine, saw a horrifying array of medical conditions resulting from use of machinery or exposure to toxic compounds, including bizarre behavior among hat workers from exposure to mercury, nerve damage among bathtub enamelers exposed to high levels of lead, "dead fingers" among workers who regularly used jackhammers, and extreme psychoses among people in the rayon industry resulting from daily exposure to carbon disulfide.

Many of these problems, particularly those resulting from chemical exposure, are considerably less than they were in past years, primarily because of legislation enforcing workplace safety. However, occupational hazards are still a concern, and employees in all fields, no matter how mundane, must constantly monitor their workplace environment to make sure they are safe.

One of the most important ongoing occupational concerns is trauma resulting from workplace accidents. Despite safety regulations, trauma still accounts for more than 10,000 occupational deaths a year, reports the National Safety Council. And according to the National Safe Workplace Institute, occupational diseases still claim tens of thousands of lives every year—despite increasingly stringent workplace safety regulations.

The number of nonfatal workplace injuries and illnesses is also remarkably high. The U.S. Department of Labor's Bureau of Labor Statistics reports that nearly half of all injuries sustained on the job are of such severity that the injured workers have to restrict or lose work time, resulting in millions of lost work days and costing industry equal amounts in lost man hours and productivity.

Occupational hazards are as unique and numerous as the jobs themselves, note health specialists. Many professions require contact with chemicals or compounds that may result in illness or an allergic reaction if not handled properly; other professions are rife with illness-causing mental stress. And, of course, everyone is aware of the repetitive-motion disorders suffered by workers whose jobs require them to perform the same repetitive activities all day long, such as data processors, butchers, and assembly-line workers.

Diagnosing work-related illness can be problematic for a couple of reasons. First, a lot of time can pass between exposure and the outbreak of symptoms, making it difficult to identify the true culprit. And second, many workplace illnesses mimic more common disorders, including cold and flu. As a result, workers may suffer for days, weeks, and even longer before making the association between work and poor health—if it's made at all.

Workplace Hazards

Occupational health experts typically divide workplace hazards into four distinct categories:

- Chemical agents, which can affect health through touch, ingestion, or inhaling
- Physical agents, such as noise or vibration (both of which can afflict industrial and construction workers)
- Biological agents, such as bacteria and viruses, which are a particular threat to healthcare workers such as doctors, nurses, and laboratory technicians
- Muscle strains and injury from using poorly designed equipment, maintaining an awkward position, and performing repetitive motions

Of course, home owners face similar risks while doing the occasional home repair, cleaning, and so on, but the men and women whose occupations expose them to hazardous substances and situations have it much worse because their exposure occurs daily. The result is cumulative toxicity. Following is a review of the most common workplace hazards. How many of them are affecting *your* health?

Chemical Hazards

Exposure to hazardous chemicals may occur as a result of your job, and you may not even know it. Take police target instructors, for example. Common sense and basic precautions may prevent them from being accidentally shot, but they are still at risk of lead exposure. The reason? Bullets are made of lead, and every time a bullet is fired, lead dust and fumes are released into the air, where they can be inhaled. Over a long period of time, exposure can be substantial. Those most at risk are instructors who work at indoor firing ranges, because there are few effective ways to cleanse the air.

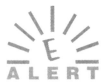
ALERT

Skin ailments are one of the most common work-related complaints. In fact, they are inherent in almost every profession, from health care, to food preparation, to office work. Workers who engage in what's known as "wet work"—that is, placing their hands in water throughout the day—are most at risk. Skin problems result when constant exposure to water, solvents, and various chemicals strip away the skin's protective oil surface, leaving the skin vulnerable to irritation. The regular use of a hand moisturizer can help.

Indeed, the chances of you being exposed to at least one potentially hazardous chemical over the course of your workday is pretty good. Of the 100,000 chemicals known to be harmful to human health, more than 10,000 can be found in the workplace.

The effects of chemical hazards on human health are numerous and potentially serious. For example, some compounds, such as asbestos and silica, can result in respiratory disease and even lung cancer if inhaled. Exposure to other chemicals, such as heavy metals, can impair the blood's ability to absorb and transport oxygen, cause rashes or allergic reactions, or damage the nervous system, kidneys, or liver. Following are more detailed accounts of the most potentially dangerous chemicals commonly found in various occupations.

Carbon monoxide

This odorless, colorless gas binds to hemoglobin in red blood cells far more strongly than oxygen, resulting in less oxygen getting to the brain and other organs. It is commonly produced by coal-burning furnaces, internal combustion engines, and, in far larger quantities, certain other industrial processes. Anyone who works in an enclosed environment with idling engines, such as garage and toll booth workers, are at high risk of carbon monoxide exposure.

Solvents

These carbon-containing liquids dissolve organic solids and are used in a wide variety of occupations. Because they are liquids that emit fumes, they can enter the body through the skin or through the lungs and damage everything from the kidneys to the nervous system. Anyone who works with solvents—and that's a lot of people—should make sure that their work environment is very well ventilated and that they wear protective clothing, including gloves, and, if necessary, a respirator.

Lead

We just can't seem to escape this dangerous heavy metal, which presents an occupational hazard to all who work in smelting operations, radiator repair, battery manufacturing, and building construction. Exposure usually occurs through the inhalation of lead fumes or vapor and is often cumulative. Proper ventilation and protective gear are essential when working with lead.

Mercury

Knowledge of the extreme toxicity of this heavy metal goes back to the ancient Egyptians, who would let only slaves and convicts mine it. Mercury is now rarely used in thermometers and was banned in 1990 as an ingredient in house paint, but it is still commonly used in a variety of industrial processes, including the manufacture of pesticides, electrical components, medical supplies, and dental amalgam. Good ventilation and protective gear are essential when working with mercury.

Physical Hazards

Physical hazards encompass much more than straining your back lifting a heavy box or having something fall on you. Depending on your occupation, physical hazards can range from ear-splitting noise, to high levels of radiation, to stifling heat. Following is a quick rundown.

Noise

In addition to damaging your ears and causing hearing impairment, chronic exposure to high levels of noise can also result in a number of serious physical ailments, often from related stress. Vibration, which often accompanies noise, can also cause serious injury, including a circulatory disorder known as Raynaud's phenomenon, or white finger syndrome. Individuals who encounter noise regularly as part of their job, such as airline mechanics and construction workers, should always wear earplugs or other protection.

Radiation

This is a word that frightens a lot of people, and it should. Regular exposure to radiation can have a cumulative effect resulting in very serious health issues. Health care workers are at particular risk due to X-rays and the frequent use of radioactive medical materials, but seemingly innocuous professions such as construction and manufacturing may also put workers at risk of exposure.

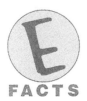

FACTS

How safe is your workplace? According to experts, in terms of relative risk, you are 1.9 times more likely to die from an occupational disease than from diabetes and twice as likely to die from a work-related accident than in a fire or by drowning.

One problem that workers may not be aware of is exposure to nonionizing radiation produced by electric and magnetic fields. The health issues related to nonionizing radiation are still being debated, but workers whose jobs require them to be around extra-low-frequency fields–for example, electricians—should at least be aware.

Temperature extremes

Many occupations require employees to work in conditions of extreme cold or heat, and these circumstances can have an adverse affect on health. Temperature extremes, as well as dramatic fluctuations in humidity, are also known to increase accident risk, so extra caution should be taken. The obvious solution is to dress properly for the job. If your job requires you to spend extended periods in extreme cold, such as packing meat or stocking frozen items in a grocery, make sure you wear a thick coat, gloves, a hat, and boots. If heat is the problem, dress as lightly as the job will allow and drink plenty of fluids throughout the day. In both situations, take frequent breaks to warm up or cool down. On the plus side, you should acclimate to the temperature extreme relatively quickly.

Biological Hazards

Biological hazards can be present both indoors and outdoors. Indoor hazards include concentrations of mold, fungi, and bacteria in office air conditioning systems or drinking water; outdoor hazards include biting or stinging insects and poisonous plants.

The various microscopic critters that can take up residence inside a building can cause some very serious health problems, including allergic reactions, rashes, colds, influenza, and even Legionnaire's disease, which is a form of pneumonia. Most cases of so-called "sick building syndrome" are the result of mold, fungi, or bacteria, though health problems may also result from chemical fumes, especially if a building is shut tight. And, of course, people who work with or encounter dangerous organisms as part of their jobs, such as health care workers and biological researchers, are also at risk, particularly if safety precautions are not enforced. Work-related hazards for this population range from a simple cold, to tuberculosis, to AIDS from an accidental needle prick.

Farmers, forest rangers, and others whose jobs require them to work outdoors also face a host of biological hazards, ranging from stinging insects, to poisonous plants, to dangerous or diseased animals. Ticks and mosquitoes are of special concern because of the many parasitic diseases they can spread, including Lyme disease, Rocky Mountain spotted fever, and viral encephalitis. As a result, anyone who works amid fields, forests, or wooded areas should take special precautions, including wearing protective clothing and the use of insect repellents.

Home owners are also at risk of biological hazards. Bacteria, mold, and fungi can flourish in a home air conditioning system as well as a commercial system, and mosquitoes and ticks can also cause serious health problems. Home owners also risk infectious diseases from their pets, such as toxoplasmosis, which can be contracted from mishandling feces and poses a serious threat to pregnant women. And if they're not careful, bird fanciers may contract psittacosis, a pulmonary disease linked to the bacteria found in bird feces.

Ergonomic Hazards

Who would have thought that merely sitting at your desk, doing your job, could be hazardous to your health? And yet, tens of thousands of office workers and others are afflicted with physical complaints as a result of stylish but poorly designed chairs, improperly tilted or placed computer screens, and other ergonomic problems.

How you sit, how long you sit, and what you do at your desk can all have an adverse effect on your body. When our alignment is off or we're forced to work in an odd position, it places strain on our muscles, tendons, and ligaments. The result can be inflamed tendons, back and joint pain, and even nerve damage.

Repetitive motion disorders are one of the most common ergonomic complaints and afflict a wide array of occupations. Very often, however, these problems can be corrected simply by giving the body greater support and making a movement more natural. For example, people who use a computer all day have found that chronic wrist pain disappears when they place a wrist support in front of the keyboard and that neck and head pain can be alleviated simply by tilting the screen up or down slightly. An ergonomic keyboard is also very helpful.

If you feel sore and achy at the end of every workday, your problem could be ergonomic. Ask your employer to have your work site evaluated by an ergonomic specialist (many insurance companies will pay for it) and heed their expert advice. It's also a good idea to take a brief break at least once an hour, particularly if your job requires rapid and repetitive motion.

Are Your Dental Fillings Poisoning You?

There has been a lot of debate in recent years regarding the impact amalgam fillings can have our health—if, indeed, they have any effect at all. Some dentists believe that the mercury and silver used to create amalgam fillings, which have been in use for decades, can result in a host of health and immune problems. However, the majority of dental authorities, including the American Dental Association (ADA), maintain that they are perfectly safe.

Whom should you believe?

One of the primary concerns among some researchers is that the mercury used in making amalgam fillings can result in neurological problems, including the onset of Alzheimer's disease. And chewing can release trace amounts of mercury vapor from amalgam fillings. However, there is no direct evidence that the amount of vapor exceeds the acceptable OSHA standard for mercury or that it produces any adverse health effects.

A recent Canadian study called for limits on the number of amalgam fillings in children and adults, but the ADA disagrees with many findings from that report. In a position statement, the ADA noted the following:

- Scientific evidence does not exist to warrant the wholesale removal of amalgam fillings.
- Although removal of existing amalgam fillings may, in some individuals, have positive effects, at this time substantial experimental evidence does not exist to confirm those positive effects. (Note: Current ADA ethics policy states that dentists commit an unethical act when they remove serviceable amalgam fillings for the sole purpose of curing some health disorder.)
- Although there is no evidence that dental amalgams contribute to immunological, neurological, or kidney disease in human populations,

there is some evidence that mercury exposure from all sources is of more significance to individuals with those problems than to the general population.

Should you have your amalgam fillings removed? Probably not—especially if you are experiencing no serious health problems. However, if you are worried, ask your physician to order a standard test for mercury in your urine. If the amount of mercury proves to be excessive (that is, over 25 micrograms per gram of creatinine), you should look into possible causes.

There are also potential dental hazards to having amalgam fillings removed just as a precaution. The integrity of the tooth can be damaged, and the removal process can release more mercury vapor than if you left your fillings alone.

Environmental Hazards and the Nervous System

All systems in the human body are vulnerable to environmental hazards such as toxic chemicals, but the nervous system is at special risk for some very important reasons:

- Neurons normally cannot regenerate once they are lost, unlike other types of cells.
- Nerve-cell loss and other changes to the nervous system occur progressively during the later years of life. As a result, toxic damage may occur simultaneously with aging.
- Many neurotoxic chemicals are easily able to cross the blood-brain barrier, causing damage to sensitive regions of the brain.
- Toxic chemicals often interfere with the nervous system's sensitive electro-chemical balance, upsetting the balance necessary for the proper communication of information throughout the body.

CHAPTER **8**

Social Support Systems

Man is a social creature by nature. While we enjoy our own space, it's important that we live and interact and connect with others—family, close friends, neighbors, acquaintances, co-workers, and even strangers. Studies have shown that losing these social connections through illness, relocation, or other causes can have a detrimental effect on our physical and emotional well-being and, thus, on how rapidly and how well we age. In short, social support plays a tremendous role in keeping us young and vital.

The Importance of Social Connections

Our need for social connections is not a new phenomenon. In fact, it's likely the reason why we succeeded as a species. During the earliest days of human existence, it became clear that there was safety and survival in numbers. A single man could spend nearly all of his waking hours hunting for food and very often have little to show for it, but a group of men, working together, could stalk and kill large prey that would provide food for several days. Groups also provided protection from larger predators and marauding invaders. As a result, loose groups of primitive humans banded together to form organized tribes, which eventually led to collectives, towns, and cities.

This primitive social interaction was important for physical survival. That's still true today; collectively we provide food, goods, and services for the survival and comfort of everyone. But more important are the emotional and psychological benefits that come from human communication and interaction. Being with friends and loved ones makes us feel good emotionally, and this, in turn, benefits our health. Indeed, social contact is vital to our development in almost every area.

The definition of social contact or social support varies among people and organizations but is generally considered to be the belief among individuals that they are cared for, loved, and part of a network of mutual obligations. This support system is instilled and confirmed by caring communication with family, friends, and others and has been shown to protect us from a wide variety of stress-related physical and mental conditions ranging from arthritis to depression. Studies have also shown that people with strong social support require less pain medication following surgery, recover more rapidly, and take better care of themselves following illness or hospitalization.

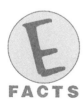

FACTS

Studies show that the risk of death is two to four times greater among people with diminishing social contact compared to those with strong connections to family and friends, even after factoring in such variables as age, race, and physical health.

The benefits of human contact and social support start from the day we're born. There's no question that babies who are frequently hugged, kissed, and loved by their families develop much better than children who grow up without this kind of loving family support.

However, the need for human connectedness does not end with childhood. It's something that we carry with us throughout our lives and that can affect our mental and physical health at any age. The elderly, in particular, are vulnerable to social isolation, a situation that can sap the very life out of a person who just months before was active and vibrant and alert. Health care practitioners speak often of the "widower effect," in which one spouse, most typically the male, dies within days or weeks of the other—even though he was, up until that time, in excellent health. This most often occurs among couples who were married for many, many years and proves the necessity and value of loving and being loved. Without it, we can literally lose the will to live.

The simple fact is that we need contact with others in order to survive. Chronic loneliness can be damaging and even deadly, while a life rich with friends and family can actually help us live longer.

In this chapter, we will look at the roles of family, marriage, friends, and pets in staying healthy and aging well. We will also take a close look at the benefits of spirituality and prayer, as well as volunteering and coping with life in the face of tragedy.

How Social Support Keeps Us Healthy

The influence of social support on our health has been confirmed by both anecdotal evidence and clinical research. It is no longer just theory; it is accepted scientific fact. We NEED strong social support to stay both mentally and physically healthy, and the changes in our health when we don't get it can be both quick and devastating.

But how does social connectedness actually help us stay healthy? What is it about being with close family and friends that does us good? Let's take a quick look at some of the benefits of a strong support system.

1. Strong social support encourages healthy living and promotes prompt medical care. Our friends and family look out for us, just as we look out for them, and often become deeply involved when we get sick. Their concern encourages us to seek medical care when necessary, and we recover faster as a result.

2. Friends and family are often impromptu "doctors," directly caring for us when we get sick. Without this assistance, we might stay sick longer or become increasingly ill.

3. Our circle of close family and friends encourages a certain degree of conformity. Very often, this includes conforming to a relatively healthful lifestyle. For example, if few of our friends smoke or drink, we are less likely to smoke or drink. Similarly, if the majority of our friends and family engage in a healthful activity, such as golf or tennis, we too are likely to pursue that activity.

4. Friendship and loving support can actually boost our immune system, making us more resistant to illness. Positive emotions can actually stimulate our body to prevent or fight illness, a phenomenon known as the mind-body connection.

A number of studies have found that strong social support provides long-term health benefits as well as short-term improvement. Married people, for example, have been found to live longer than unmarried people, and those who actively participate in an organized religion tend to live longer than those who do not. In the long run, it seems, ongoing, positive social support can work wonders in helping us live to a ripe old age.

Not all social support is conducive to good health, however. Very often, good intentions can actually worsen a medical problem by causing someone to postpone medical treatment ("I wouldn't worry about that rash; it'll probably get better on its own.") or advising the use of alternative therapies over established medical care. And just as social support can encourage healthful conformity, so too can peer pressure promote unhealthy habits, such as smoking, excessive alcohol consumption, or drug use—especially among impressionable young people.

FACTS

One of the most important aspects of living a long, full life is starting off healthy and strong. But researchers in England have found that many babies enter the world weighing less than they should and with a host of other problems simply because their mothers do not receive sufficient social support during pregnancy. Women with several types of support from different sources during pregnancy have higher birth weight infants.

The Role of Family

As noted, close family ties are important for proper mental and physical health. There's a phenomenon known as "skin hunger," in which people who are socially isolated for whatever reason desperately yearn for the comforting touch of another human being. This is particularly true of infants who are abandoned and forced to develop and grow with little physical or mental connectedness.

The importance of family love in health and development was demonstrated by Harvard researchers who bred a strain of mice lacking a gene believed instrumental to learning and memory. The new strain showed no outward defects until they bred and bore young; their litters seemed healthy at first, but soon died. However, when their babies were removed at birth and raised by normal mice, they flourished. The problem? The mice lacking the learning and memory gene ignored their young. They didn't attack them or harm them but simply didn't care for them. They didn't go out of their way to keep them warm, or round them up when they wandered away, or help them nurse. In short, they showed no parental concern at all, and as a result, their young failed to flourish and died.

Humans and mice are decidedly different creatures, but the moral of this study—that a lack of nurturing care and physical contact can have a strong adverse effect on growth, development, and overall health—is true for almost all animals that bring forth living young. We are dependent on family ties for survival, and when we don't get it, the consequences can be devastating.

When it comes to aging, the role of family is varied and deeply important. A close-knit family provides unconditional love and support, which helps members deal with stressful life events such as the death of a friend or loved one, the loss of a job, relocation, the birth of a child, divorce, or serious illness. This factor alone makes family a vital component in our anti-aging regimen.

Family support through role modeling and encouragement also plays an important role in maintaining proper health. Examples include mothers pushing their children (and spouse) to eat better, exercise more, and be careful when out of the house; fathers engaging in recreational sports with their sons and daughters; and siblings being watchful of each other at school and at play. By promoting healthful living, our families encourage us to live better and thus extend our potential lifespan. They may not say, "Eat your broccoli so you'll live longer," but the result is the same.

FACTS

The healing power of humor is not a new phenomenon. In the early 1300s, surgeon Henri de Mondesville noted: "Let the surgeon take care to regulate the whole regimen of the patient's life for joy and happiness, allowing his relatives and special friends to cheer him, and by having someone tell him jokes."

In addition, family connections help keep us young by providing interaction between young and old. This concept is wonderfully illustrated in Lynn Johnston's daily comic strip *For Better or for Worse*, which features an ongoing story line in which Ellie Patterson's father comes to live with Ellie and her family following the death of his wife. The social support offered by his family helps Grandpa come to grips with his grief; it also shows him that he is still needed. At the same time, Grandpa's relationship with his young granddaughter, April, opens up a world of opportunity for them both. April helps Grandpa feel young, and Grandpa shows April the simple pleasures in life, such as learning how to play the harmonica.

Without even trying, young children have a remarkable capacity for energizing and maintaining the youth of older family members. They make us laugh, they make us think, and they remind us constantly of why it's important that we stay young and vital, even as we age chronologically. Not surprisingly, many older Americans attribute their longevity and youthful vigor to doing volunteer work with children, such as assisting in classrooms and youth centers or participating in mentoring programs.

The healthful benefits of regular interaction between younger and older family members works both ways. Young people help keep aging family members vital through their youthful enthusiasm and lust for life, while older family members aid children and grandchildren by imparting to them the wisdom they have learned through living. Advice and counsel from someone who has been there and understands well the various pitfalls of adolescence and young adulthood can go a long way toward ensuring that a boy or girl grows up healthy, motivated, and eager to learn.

Finally, family support plays an especially important role as members grow older. We've all heard the horror stories of elderly parents being dumped in nursing homes or hospital emergency rooms because their families couldn't (or wouldn't) care for them any longer. However, the vast majority of Americans go to extraordinary lengths to care for their aging family members. They care for them at home when they become ill, and when they can no longer do that, they look for the very best institutional accommodations they can afford, visit their loved ones often, and fret that they can't do more. This kind of loving support can go a long way toward extending the life expectancy of older family members and dramatically reduces the physical and mental deterioration often attributed to social isolation.

The Role of Marriage

The support one receives from a loving personal relationship with a significant other—traditionally in the form of marriage—has long been recognized as beneficial to one's well-being. Statistically, married people live longer than those who do not marry and experience better health overall than single people.

The reasons for this are many. For one thing, married couples traditionally provide each other with a huge amount of social support in the form of love and companionship. In a strong, reciprocal marriage, this can have a very strong influence on physical and mental health and, in the process, help reduce the effects of aging.

In many cases, married couples benefit each other healthwise through support and encouragement. For example, a nonsmoking spouse may help his or her smoking partner kick the habit, or the more active member may encourage the other to exercise more. This doesn't occur through nagging; that's a form of communication that usually does more harm than good. Instead, we're talking about the kind of support and encouragement that comes from wanting what's best for our life partner and doing what we can to make it a reality. Living by example is one of the best ways to help someone overcome less than healthy habits, and the close proximity of marriage often enables this to happen.

A good marriage is also an effective way to combat the stress we encounter in our daily lives—stress, for example, from heavy traffic, angry bosses, and unbearable deadlines. Married people are able to vent their fears and frustrations to a caring ear and receive positive, stress-reducing feedback. The result is far fewer stress-related ailments. Single people, on the other hand, must deal with stress on their own, which in some cases means turning to liquor or drugs.

The physical and mental benefits of married sex is also an important consideration. Of course, sex isn't only for married couples; single people can enjoy loving, satisfying sexual relationships as well. However, for many married couples, romance and sex become important ways of demonstrating an often unspoken depth of love that supports and heals and nurtures on a number of different levels. Through sex, many married couples often bond in a way that singles can't understand or take advantage of. It becomes a form of unspoken communication capable of carrying couples through stressful times and, in so doing, protecting them from a wide variety of health problems.

The Role of Friends

One of the best things you can do for your health—and to control the aging process—is have plenty of good friends. Enduring friendship is one of the most important components of a strong social support network, and without it we set ourselves up for a myriad of problems.

In years past, researchers didn't want to believe that social factors actually played a role in our biological health, but ever-increasing amounts of data show a direct correlation between strong interpersonal relationships and human health, particularly the role of friendship in maintaining a strong immune system. For example, studies have found that people with a lot of friends have one-quarter to one-half the risk of lonely people of dying prematurely and that women with a strong friendship base are both less likely to develop deadly cancers and far more likely to survive when cancer does occur. Even less serious health issues appear to be influenced by friendship. One study found that problems related to menopause are much more common among women who lack a strong circle of friends. Other female health issues, such as PMS, menstrual cramps, and complications during pregnancy, also appear to be more common among women with little social support.

How does friendship keep us healthy? Well, as noted earlier, it often encourages us to conform to a more healthful lifestyle. If our friends like to exercise, chances are that we'll join them; if they put a strong emphasis on nutrition, so will we—at least to a certain degree. Our circle of friends can be constant reminders of what we need to do right.

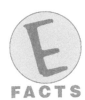
FACTS

Many physical therapy and rehabilitation clinics are incorporating dogs and other animals into their regimens as a way of making patient recovery faster and more enjoyable. At the Rehabilitation Institute of Chicago, for example, a stroke victim with limited use of an arm might work to improve strength and movement by combing a Labrador retriever, and a head injury patient might boost his memory skills by giving a list of vocal commands to a poodle. Sessions also provide patients with valuable social contact and emotional support, say therapists.

Like marriage, friendship also helps us cope with stress. One of the most important ways is by stimulating a feeling of relaxation. This is extremely beneficial because relaxation reduces stress, which is good for the heart and other systems, and boosts the immune system, which helps ward off illness. Whether it's chatting with friends over a couple of cold ones at the local diner or catching up on the week's events over dinner at home, the relationship we have with our friends induces a state of calm and contentment. We can also vent to friends in ways that we can't with others. They understand us and want the best for us. They encourage us, support us, and are happy for our successes.

In addition, friendship also gives us peace of mind. It's reassuring to know that we have a strong social network, that our friends are a quick phone call away should we ever need them. People who live alone or who have few friends, perhaps because of forced relocation, often lack this peace of mind because their support system is extremely limited. Who will help them if they become ill? Who can they talk to when they have problems? These are important considerations that, if negatively dwelled upon long enough, can actually make us sick.

Most of us carry a certain number of close friends throughout our entire lives. Faces may come and go, but the depth of our friendships typically remains the same. However, our circle of friends can be devastated by a great many life events. A family move, for example, can immediately separate us from friends we've had for decades. And many seniors suddenly find established friendships torn asunder when they are forced to move into a nursing home or retirement community due to failing health.

However, many times a move into a retirement community can actually have the reverse effect; without even trying, an individual may find himself or herself going from no friends to many within the course of just a few days. Retirement communities, which are much more conducive to an active lifestyle than traditional nursing homes, encourage interaction between residents, and most residents go out of their way to make new arrivals feel welcome. As a result, it's not uncommon for someone whose functional ability was debilitated by loneliness and isolation to suddenly revitalize and find that life is again worth living.

If your circle of friends is somewhat limited and you would like more, there are many things you can do, including the following:

- Join an organization based on a shared interest. If you're a veteran, for example, consider joining the VFW. If you love reading, join a book discussion group.

- Do volunteer work. In addition to meeting new people and making new friends, you'll find that volunteering actually improves your health.

- Make a concerted attempt to meet your neighbors. In today's somewhat isolationist society, it's not uncommon for families to live next door to each other for years yet never really know each other. If this is the case with you, invite your neighbors to a "meet and greet" party and find out what you have in common. Perhaps your new best friend is right across the street!

- Explore your spiritual side. Most churches and synagogues host socials and other events so that members can get to know each other better.

- If you're athletic, consider joining a team or group sport such as baseball, softball, golf, or tennis.

- Consider joining a support group if something in your life is overwhelming you, such as the loss of a loved one, an ongoing family crisis such as a parent with Alzheimer's disease, or the diagnosis of a serious illness. Friendship and support can go a long way toward helping us overcome personal adversity. The worst thing you can do is hold it in and try to deal with it alone.

Whenever possible, do what you can to stay in touch with distant friends, especially those you've known for many years. Lifelong friendships are especially important and should never be abandoned if possible. At the very least, call friends in other states once a week just to stay in touch and provide support if needed. Thanks to inexpensive long-distance telephone plans and even less expensive computer e-mail, there's no excuse for letting a friendship go by the wayside.

The Role of Pets

Pets can contribute tremendously to our social support and, thus, to our longevity. Numerous studies have been conducted regarding the healthful benefits of pet ownership, and the results have been universally positive. Without question, having loving animals in our lives enriches in a number of different ways.

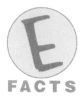

A great many American presidents have kept dogs as pets, and very often these animals have played a vital role in reducing stress and anxiety during troubling times. A Welsh terrier named Charlie, for example, helped John Kennedy deal with the Cuban missile crisis, perhaps one of the most frightening periods of the 1960s.

One of the most consistent findings among the many studies evaluating the beneficial role of pets in our lives is that they provide an important measure of stress relief. Simply petting or playing with our favorite pet, whether it's a dog, cat, hamster, or canary, stimulates the production of calming chemicals within the brain and helps us relax. Watching fish in an aquarium has a similar calming effect.

The calming influence of small animals is so effective that many doctors recommend daily pet play as therapy for their patients who are under a lot of stress either at work or at home. Fifteen minutes of tossing a yarn ball to some frolicsome kittens is a wonderful and inexpensive way to shed the stress of a hard day at the office. If you're not a cat person, playing fetch with your dog is equally beneficial. The point is to spend time with your pet, whatever the species, and enjoy its company. Talk to it. Pet it. Scratch it behind the ears. Bask in the glow of the pet-owner bond and feel the anxiety melt away. Even the most stressful day is no match for a puppy that's so happy to see you that its tail is a blur.

Pets, particularly dogs and cats, also contribute to our social support by providing unconditional love. This is particularly important to people who may have lost much of their inner circle due to the loss of a spouse or separation from family. Lacking human friends with whom to share their emotions, they often turn to their faithful animals for solace and support.

Very frequently, pet owners will say that they receive more love from their animals than they do from the humans in their lives. This may be somewhat of an exaggeration, but in many cases, it's not much of one. People being people, we are sometimes unintentionally hurtful, indifferent, or selfish to those we care most about. But these characteristics are almost never seen in dogs or cats. It's easy to give our pets human emotions and characteristics, but when all is said and done, very often it really is our pets who show us the greatest love, affection, and gratitude. For a great many people, this loving bond is a driving force; without it, they would wither and die. So never discount the love you receive from your pets, and always do what you can to reciprocate.

Pets also improve our lives by encouraging us to exercise. In fact, for many people with sedentary jobs, walking the dog is the only daily physical activity they get. But even that little bit of exercise is good, say doctors. So in this small way, our pets are striving to help us live longer.

A brisk walk with your dog twice a day or a game of fetch with a stick or a Frisbee can provide a good workout for the both of you. If you're a cat person, a game of "chase around the house" can easily get your heart beating a little quicker. And some people even include their cats in their daily workout, using the cat as weight for arm curls and other exercises. Of course, only an especially docile cat would let you use it as an exercise device, but if your pet doesn't mind being handled, it's certainly worth a try.

Playtime with your pet will benefit you body and soul. The actual physical activity improves strength and endurance, while the time spent with your pet strengthens the special bond the two of you share, a bond that can boost self-esteem and make you feel both needed and loved. The result: Less stress, greater vitality, a stronger immune system, and improved longevity.

The Role of Spirituality

Can faith in a higher power help us live longer? It's a controversial concept that has sparked much debate within the medical and theological communities, but there is some very strong evidence that spirituality (in whatever form works best for you) can have a very positive impact on your physical and mental health, and thus on your longevity.

For example, Harold Koenig, M.D., director of the Duke University Center for the Study of Religion, Spirituality, and Health, studied eighty-seven profoundly depressed patients at Duke University Medical Center. He found that those who considered themselves very spiritual recovered 70 percent faster than those who didn't.

In a separate study involving 1,700 people, Dr. Koenig compared immune system factors in those who attended religious services (even if it was just once a month) with those who never attended religious services. His findings? Those who attended religious services had noticeably stronger immune systems. Are you finding all of this interesting? Let's take a look at a few more findings.

- A study at the California Public Health Foundation in Berkeley found that women who go to church at least once a week have a significantly lower chance of dying prematurely than do women who never attend religious services. The finding is significant because the study also took into account health factors such as smoking, drinking, amount of exercise, and weight.
- Heart surgery patients who said they received strength and comfort from their religion were three times more likely to survive than those who did not, report researchers at the Dartmouth-Hitchcock Medical Center in Lebanon, New Hampshire.
- A study of 113 women at the University of North Carolina in Greensboro found a strong link between lower blood pressure and strong religious beliefs—even after factoring in such things as weight, diet, and other lifestyle issues.
- A study of nearly 92,000 men and women by researchers at Johns Hopkins University in Baltimore found that weekly church-goers died 50 percent less often from heart disease, emphysema, and suicide, and 74 percent less often from cirrhosis than people who did not attend church.

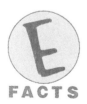

FACTS

During the 1800s, it was commonly believed that people's personality could be interpreted by "reading" the bumps on their head. This pseudoscience, known as phrenology, was eventually dismissed as quackery—but not before a great many phrenologists made a fortune reading the skulls of a gullible public.

Not too long ago, researchers who wanted to examine the healthful potential of spirituality would have been laughed out of the profession.

Today, numerous respected institutions are studying the impact of faith on health and longevity, with some very interesting results. More than 300 studies have found that people who embrace religious faith are healthier than nonbelievers and far less likely to die prematurely from any cause. Deep religious faith has also been found to speed recovery from surgery and even mental illness. The question remains: How does faith help us stay healthy?

- Belief in God and participation in an organized religion provides hope and solace during troubled times. Without this grounding force, life's problems can result in overwhelming stress which in turn can have an adverse affect on our health.
- Religious people tend to take better care of themselves in all aspects of their lives. They are less likely than nonreligious people to smoke or drink to excess, and more likely to exercise regularly, take their medicines, and wear safety belts when driving.
- Religious faith usually involves strong community ties, which can have a positive effect on our physical and mental well-being. Most religious people view their place of worship as family, which promotes strong feelings of connection and purpose. Religious people tend to take care of each other, praying for those who are ill and maintaining strong social ties during times of crisis.
- Human beings are genetically programmed to believe in a higher power, which in turn promotes a more healthful attitude, feeling, and lifestyle.

It must be noted that simply claiming to be religious probably won't have any beneficial effect on your health and longevity. The good comes from practicing heartfelt religious beliefs, rather than spending an hour in church every Sunday on the off chance that it'll help you live longer.

Of course, it's never too late to bring spirituality into your life. Approach religion with an open mind (and heart) and check out a variety of faiths if you don't already belong to one. Many people find that the religion in which they grew up really isn't the faith that benefits them the most as adults. It also helps to talk with clerics about the specific tenets of their denominations. By learning all you can about a specific religion, you can determine how well it fits into your basic feelings regarding spirituality.

FACTS

In 1967, a South African heart surgeon named Christian Barnard made medical history by performing the first human heart transplant. The recipient was fifty-five-year-old Louis Washkansky, who was slowly dying of heart disease. The donor was twenty-five-year-old Denise Darvall, who had been killed in a car accident. Barnard, supported by a team of thirty assistants, gave Washkansky a new lease on life, albeit a short one; Washkansky contracted pneumonia and died just eighteen days after receiving the new organ. However, the surgery demonstrated the viability of transplanting the human heart and paved the way for a new era in organ transplantation.

The Healthful Benefits of Prayer

Now that we've discussed the role of spirituality on longevity, lets take a look at the specific healing power of prayer. As amazing as it may seem, numerous studies have shown that prayer really can help the sick and ailing—even at a distance, and even if a person doesn't know he or she is being prayed for. In addition, frequent prayer also appears to benefit those who do the praying. It's a thought provoking aspect of spirituality and health care that begs for more research.

Dr. Herbert Benson, a researcher at Harvard Medical School and one of the first people to popularize the mind-body connection, showed a distinct relationship between prayer and health. In various studies, Benson concluded that frequent praying can do everything from lowering high blood pressure to easing cancer pain.

Other studies have drawn similar conclusions. In a Duke University study addressing the issue of posthospitalization depression, researchers analyzed 1,000 hospital patients and found that those who drew on religious practices—including prayer—were able to cope far better than those who did not draw strength from their religious beliefs.

Most astounding, however, is the apparent effectiveness of intercessory prayer, in which the sick are prayed for from a distance, and often without their knowledge. In one revealing research project, cardiologist Randolph Byrd studied 393 patients admitted to the coronary care unit at San Francisco General Hospital. In a randomized, double-blind approach, some of the patients were prayed for by members of home-prayer groups and others were not. The results: Those who were prayed for required fewer drugs and spent less time on ventilators. They also recovered more quickly and did better overall than those who received only medical care.

Studies on living, nonhuman subjects have had similar results. Plants that were prayed for grew taller, yeast was more resistant to toxic substances, and test-tube bacteria multiplied faster.

One thing is evident in all of these studies—healing prayer involves empathy and compassion. Intent is vital. Merely uttering the words will not have the same effect as praying with the heartfelt hope that those being prayed for will get better quickly.

Can prayer help us live longer? In a roundabout way, yes. Being prayed for by others and doing the same in return can be a strong aspect of social support for many people. It can help us get through periods of stress, hardship, or tragedy and help us maintain our mental well-being. Through all of that, we receive a wide variety of physical benefits. All that is required is sincerity.

Charity and Volunteerism: The Importance of Community Involvement

Despite the bad news that bombards us daily from the front page of the newspaper and the talking heads on the evening news, human beings are, overall, charitable and compassionate creatures. We willingly go out of our way to help others in need and, in so doing, help ourselves in a variety of interesting ways.

Studies have shown that people who regularly volunteer their time and services to those in need demonstrate better health and greater longevity than those who don't. Helping others improves our mood, reduces the effects of stress, and boosts our immune system. But in order

to enjoy the healthful benefits of volunteerism, you actually have to participate. Simply writing a check to your favorite charity isn't enough; you need
to get out there and become physically involved.

FACTS

Scientific evidence that light to moderate consumption of alcohol can protect the heart and circulatory system should not be construed as an excuse to hit the bottle like a sailor on shore leave. Here are some facts from the National Council on Alcoholism and Drug Dependence:

- It's estimated that more than 12 million Americans show signs of alcohol abuse or dependence and that an additional 8 million show persistent, heavy drinking problems that affect or impair their health.
- Ten percent of the population consumes 50 percent of the alcohol.
- Fifty to 70 percent of alcoholics display neurological abnormalities.
- Alcoholics have thirty times the suicide rate of nondrinkers.

A growing number of Americans are discovering the pleasures of helping their fellow human being, with the fastest growing demographic being retirees. Rather than stay at home and waste away watching television, a sizable percentage of America's senior population are hitting the streets, working at churches, hospitals, nursing homes, schools, libraries, and charitable organizations. Having spent so much of their lives struggling to support themselves and their families, they now want to do what they can to help others. And they're living longer as a result.

There is tremendous satisfaction in performing charity and volunteer work, and you're never too young or too old to start. What you do, for whom, and for how long is strictly a personal decision, but it should be something close to your heart; if you're just going through the motions, you might as well stay home. Do you enjoy working with older people? Perhaps you could spend a few hours a week visiting with lonely residents at an area nursing home. If children are more your passion, schools are always in need of classroom assistants. Consult family, friends, and your clergy for some additional suggestions. You'll be doing yourself and others a world of good.

Social Support in Old Age

The importance of social support in old age cannot be underestimated. It's during this time of life when support from family, friends, and social agencies is most vital, and the lack of it can cause a serious deterioration in physical and mental health.

Many people erroneously believe that the demands for support increase with age but that the support system is ever-shrinking. Studies have found this to be untrue. In reality, the network of social support tends to remain surprisingly stable as people go through life. According to the MacArthur Foundation Study on Aging, considered one of the most comprehensive studies on aging in America, one of the most important factors in successful aging is how many supportive people we have in our "inner circle" and what kind of support they provide.

To understand this better, think of support systems as a series of ever-smaller concentric circles, sort of like an archery target, with you in the center. Those closest to you are in the innermost circle—family, best friends, clergy, and so forth. These people provide the strongest support and are extremely vital to our health and longevity; they make life worth living. The outward circles are groups of diminishing support or influence; they include acquaintances, coworkers, and so forth. These people are still important and offer valuable support in various ways, but their impact on our lives is not quite as strong as those of the innermost circle. By drawing such a chart, you can see for yourself where your greatest social support comes from and the kind of impact these individuals have on your life. This support network stays surprisingly stable throughout life for the majority of people, even into old age. Members come and go, but the support network itself stays strong and vital.

The authors of the book reporting the results of the MacArthur Foundation Study on Aging use the word *convoy* to describe the social support network we carry throughout our lives because the term conveys a sense of group protection, much like a convoy of ships during wartime. This is an apt analogy; our social support networks provide protection from loneliness by offering companionship and stability during periods of stress and change. This is particularly important during our latter years, when change becomes increasingly common—and particularly devastating. We lose spouses and other family members, long-time friends and passing acquaintances, jobs, and homes. The senior years are rife with change and instability, and it's during this period of our lives that our network of friends and loved ones becomes ever so necessary to our very survival. Without them, we would be awash in loneliness and despair, and our health would almost certainly suffer.

Studies show that the more diverse our innermost circle of social support, the better off we are. It's important that we associate with people who share our mind-set—for example, with those who think young regardless of their age—but diversity of personalities and ages is also essential. As noted, older people, in particular, benefit greatly from being with close friends who are younger than them because their vitality is contagious. We stay young by being young.

Likewise, it's important that our closest circle of friends and loved ones be positive in personality. Associating with Gloomy Gus or Depressed Dave will only bring us down and, in the long run, adversely affect our health. Psychologists call such people "toxic personalities" and suggest that they be avoided because of their potential detrimental effects. If you are surrounded by "toxic" family members, try to counter their negative influence by spending as much time as possible with more positive and helpful individuals.

According to researchers, the more that older people participate in close social relationships, the better their overall physical and mental health, and the higher their level of function. The definition of *social relationship* is broad and can include everything from daily phone chats with family to regular visits with close friends to attending church every Sunday.

The MacArthur Foundation Study on Aging revealed that the two strongest predictors of well-being among the elderly are frequency of visits with friends and frequency of attendance at organization meetings.

And the more meaningful the contribution in a particular activity, the greater the health benefit. For example, people who consider themselves spiritual or religious, attend religious services regularly, and are active within their church or synagogue appear to do better than those who simply say they are religious.

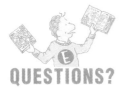

QUESTIONS?

Is it possible for older people to receive too much support?
Absolutely! And it can have a detrimental effect on their physical health and mental well-being by inhibiting the development of independent skills and self-esteem.

Problems occur when support members such as friends and family offer too much assistance to older family and friends. Constant assistance, while well intentioned, can affect how people view themselves and their ability to function on a daily basis. They may ask themselves, Am I so feeble that I really need this much help? Cognitive function, like the body's muscles and other systems, needs to be "exercised" in order to remain strong and vital, doctors note. Too much assistance can quickly reduce that vitality.

It's one thing to occasionally assist an older family member or friend when they genuinely need it, but it's quite another to do virtually everything for them in the mistaken belief that old age equals low functional ability. Unfortunately, older people who are constantly assisted in their daily living may find themselves victims of what is known as "learned helplessness." And once on that road, it's difficult to turn back.

Social Support and Mental Acuity

We've talked extensively about the physical value of social support in this book, but it's important that you also understand the extraordinary value it has in maintaining mental acuity. A lack of social support can be as devastating as disease or injury when it comes to eroding mental function.

Indeed, a life rich with friends and loved ones can be one of the best elixirs when it comes to keeping our brains strong and vital. The importance of social support was demonstrated during a recent study at a large nursing home. Residents were randomly divided into three groups and given the task of completing a jigsaw puzzle. All three of the groups were given four twenty-minute practice sessions, followed by a timed session. Members of the first group were given a lot of verbal encouragement by the experiment director during the practice sessions, members in the second group were given direct assistance, and members of the third group received neither encouragement nor assistance.

The results of the experiment were intriguing. Those in the group that received a lot of encouragement demonstrated marked improvement in both speed and proficiency in putting the puzzle together during the timed session. In other words, their mental acuity apparently improved due to the social support they received during practice. Those who were directly assisted did less well during the timed session than during practice, and those who were left alone showed no change at all.

What does this mean? Foremost, this experiment demonstrates how social support in the form of interaction and encouragement can improve cognitive function in older people. However, it also demonstrates that the support must be appropriate to the individual and what he or she wishes to accomplish, whether it's a stronger memory or improved visual-spatial skills. Daily chats about the previous night's television shows may be seen as social support, but mere conversation with friends won't improve mental tasks.

Similarly, this experiment clearly shows the importance of social support and what gerontologists call self-efficacy—that is, a person's belief that he or she can handle life's daily situations appropriately and effectively. The group that received assistance didn't do quite as well as the group that received reassurance and support; this is because assistance suggests to group members that they are incapable of doing it themselves. Too much assistance is a common phenomenon among America's elderly; family and friends complete tasks rather than let the elderly do it themselves. Sometimes this is done out of love and other times out of frustration or impatience; however, regardless of the motive, it only helps to instill a feeling of inadequacy and helplessness.

Strong self-efficacy is as important for mental skills as it is for physical skills. Older people must be able to prove to themselves through a series of successes that they can and have mastered a particular function, such as memory. Confidence is key to success, and those who don't feel confident will almost certainly fail when challenged by specific mental tasks. Social support in the form of encouragement can play a pivotal role in instilling confidence and strengthening mental acuity. This is important to remember regardless of age. If you believe that something can be done, you will find success.

Maintaining a Positive Attitude in the Face of Tragedy

No life is free of tragedy, nor should it be. Bad times help us appreciate the good and give us a clearer perspective on what constitutes a life well lived.

Unfortunately, some people encounter more tragedy than others over the course of their lives, whether it's devastating illness or injury, the loss of friends or loved ones, or missed opportunities. Recurring tragedy can have a negative impact on our mental and physical well-being and influence our longevity. Here are some tips on maintaining a positive attitude in the face of overwhelming adversity.

- *Don't hold in your emotions.* Seek solace from friends, loved ones, and support groups. A stoic attitude will not help you feel better, but comfort from loving friends will.
- *Don't hesitate to seek professional help.* There's no shame in seeing a psychologist when overwhelmed by negative life experiences. Talking with a professional will help you put such events in perspective and get on with your life.
- *Recognize the physical and mental signs of depression.* It's only natural to become depressed in the face of adversity. Often these feelings are fleeting and your good spirits return within a few days. But if depression lasts longer than two weeks, or if you feel overwhelmed by feelings of melancholy, desperation, and hopelessness to the point of self-harm or suicide, seek help at once. Nearly all depression is treatable, but you have to take the first step.

- *Don't turn to alcohol or drugs for relief.* Both are short-term solutions that ultimately do more harm than good. Far more effective strategies are available; simply ask your doctor.
- *Do continue to take care of yourself.* This means eating right and getting plenty of exercise. The latter can be particularly helpful because exercise stimulates the production of mood-altering brain chemicals.

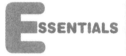

ESSENTIALS

In a recent study conducted at Duke University Medical Center, 150 study participants—all of them fifty years or older and diagnosed with depression—took one of three treatments for four months: exercise, the antidepressant Zoloft, or a combination of the two. Six months after the study, those who had been in the exercise group had significantly lower depression relapse rates than those in the Zoloft or combination groups.

Humor and Health: Living Longer Through Laughter

Reader's Digest had it right all along—laughter really is the best medicine! Numerous studies have found that facing life's adversities with humor rather than anger or fear can go a long way toward a successful resolution, as well as maintaining sound physical and mental well-being.

Humor and laughter benefit us in a wide variety of ways. For one thing, a good sense of humor provides needed stress relief. When we laugh at our problems rather than fret over them, they become less serious and thus easier to solve. Humor also improves cognitive function by keeping the mind active and encouraging creative thinking—a vital defense against age—and provides an important emotional catharsis during periods of emotional tension.

Norman Cousins was one of the first American researchers to actively promote the physical healing properties of humor. In 1979, he incorporated laughter into his treatment for ankylosing spondylitis, theorizing that if negative emotions have a negative impact on our health, then positive emotions would have a healing effect. To improve his good humor, Cousins watched funny movies and television shows, laughing his way to successful healing. During the last years of his life, Cousins established the Humor Research Task Force at the UCLA Medical School Department of Behavioral Medicine, coordinating and supporting clinical research worldwide on the healing effects of humor.

Humor not only puts us in a better mood and helps us cope with life's problems but also has a dramatic impact on the body. Researchers at Loma Linda University School of Medicine's Department of Clinical Immunology conducted numerous studies proving that laughter helps lower serum cortisol levels, increases the amount of activated T lymphocytes, increases the number and activity of natural killer cells, and increases the number of T cells that have helper/suppressor receptors. In other words, laughter helps stimulate the immune system and counters the immunosuppressive effects of stress.

Laughter also benefits the heart, improves oxygen flow to the brain, and works the muscles in the head, neck, chest, and pelvis—in much the same way as the stress reduction exercises of yoga. This helps keep muscles loose and limber and enables them to rest more easily.

So the next time illness strikes, take a couple of aspirin, drink plenty of fluids—and pop a Marx Brothers movie in the VCR. You'll soon be laughing yourself to wellness.

CHAPTER 9

Specifics for Individual Populations

Anti-aging is not a one-size-fits-all kind of thing because human beings are not one-size-fits-all creatures. There are dramatic physiological differences between the genders, which means that certain anti-aging supplements, technologies, and dietary requirements may be better suited for one sex than the other. This chapter is going to take a look at anti-aging specifics for individual populations.

Recognizing Differences

Ongoing life changes make the prospect of a simple, all-purpose anti-aging pill extremely slim. It might be possible if all human beings were exactly alike and our needs never varied from one life phase to another, but such is not the case. We change as we grow, and this must be an important consideration in all anti-aging research.

It must also be an important consideration when creating an individualized anti-aging regimen. The typical husband and wife in their mid-thirties—let's call them Bill and Sue—may be able to engage in certain anti-aging activities together, such as going to the gym for regular exercise, but the differences in their personal regimens are far greater than the similarities. Sue faces dramatic changes in physiology as she goes from puberty through her childbearing years to menopause; how she handles these changes can have an important effect on her longevity. Her physical and nutritional needs will change; she will be prone to different, more gender-based ailments; and her emotional and psychological well-being will also feel the influence. Bill's body will change, too, but in a different and less dramatic way. As a result, while their ultimate goal is the same—more healthful years to their lives—Bill and Sue will have to pursue decidedly different approaches in achieving that goal.

In this chapter, we will analyze the differences in anti-aging for men, women, children, the elderly, and those with special needs, with an emphasis on current and future health requirements. This is important because one of the greatest contributing factors to extended longevity in all populations is staying healthy throughout life. Staying healthy means doing the following:

- Eating according to our needs
- Exercising according to our abilities
- Maintaining a healthful lifestyle (i.e., avoiding harmful activities such as smoking)
- Taking advantage of anti-aging breakthroughs where safe and appropriate
- Actively seeking social support

Bottom line: An effective anti-aging regimen should be unique to you and your needs, but it should also grow and evolve as you age. Your approach twenty years from now will almost certainly be much different from your approach today, but it's never too early to start planning. The keys to success are self-awareness and continuing education.

Anti-aging and Men

Anti-aging research, it seems, has a pro-male bias. The majority of available supplements and technologies seem to favor men over other populations (with the exception of cosmeceuticals, which are more actively geared toward women), and quite a bit of anti-aging advertising seems to be focused specifically on the male consumer. It's wrong, of course, to think that the anti-aging phenomenon appeals only to men, but that's the way the industry seems to be heading. No doubt that will change dramatically in coming years as new technologies are developed with unique populations in mind.

Whether men take advantage of the anti-aging philosophies and products currently available is strictly an individual decision. Some pop pills and down elixirs as if their lives literally depend on it; others do very little when it comes to combating the aging process.

The various approaches to anti-aging, as well as the most current findings on the subject, are discussed at great length in the following chapter. There are, however, certain issues that all men should consider if they want to live to a ripe old age.

Men and Nutrition

In general, men are less concerned about the food they eat than women. To most, if it's flavorful and fills them up, then it's good food. However, the anti-aging benefits of proper nutrition are just as important to men as any other population, and the smart man must realize this if he wants to add a significant number of healthful years to his life. Following are some general tips:

- *Reduce the amount of red meat in your diet.* This will help lower your risk of serious illness later in life, including heart disease, stroke, diabetes, and certain forms of cancer. Consider alternatives such as fish and pasta. (When you do eat red meat, make sure it's lean and well cooked.)

- *Add more fresh fruits and vegetables.* They contain important anti-aging compounds, including disease-fighting antioxidants. Try to consume at least five servings every day.
- *Reduce your consumption of fatty foods, processed foods, and snack foods.* They contain very little nutrition and are packed with chemicals your body doesn't need.
- *Consume sugar and salt in moderation.* Neither adds much nutritionally, and both can cause a variety of health problems, including obesity and hypertension.
- *Limit your alcohol consumption.* One or two drinks a day can actually benefit your body, but more than that is unhealthy.
- *Take a vitamin/mineral supplement daily.* Most men do not receive the RDA of the most important nutrients from their diet, so supplementation is important.

Men and Exercise

More men are exercising today than ever before, but it's still a tiny percentage of the overall male population. Physical activity is essential to good health and a long life, yet many men spend their days sitting at a desk and are too tired to exercise by the time they finally get home.

If this sounds like you, it's time to make some changes. No one can force you to exercise, but it's almost guaranteed that you will feel better once you do. Exercise builds overall strength, increases stamina, and makes you look better physically. It also benefits your body by stimulating your immune system and keeping the heart and lungs in good working order.

For most men, the biggest obstacle to regular exercise is time, particularly if they work a standard eight-hour workday. If you find yourself in this situation, you have three "exercise windows" each day—morning, lunchtime, and after work. And you may have to try all three before determining which is best for you.

Many men find that exercising before they go to work helps energize them for the day. They arrive at work wide awake, fully pumped, and ready to face whatever challenge confronts them. Best of all, their daily exercise is over early, so they can concentrate on other matters for the rest of the day.

But if you'd rather sleep in an extra hour, perhaps a lunchtime workout is better. An increasing number of companies are realizing the employee benefits of an on-site fitness center, but if your company is still behind the times, don't worry—most cities have at least one fitness center within just a few minutes of almost anywhere. A lunchtime workout saves time and lets you return to the office invigorated. The downside: It's difficult to entertain clients when you're doing bench presses. Time can also be a concern in that it may be difficult to fit in an entire workout within the standard forty-five minutes to an hour typically allotted for lunch.

Given a choice, most men would rather exercise after work. They find that it helps them to relax after a hard day at the office, eliminates stress, and reduces their dinnertime appetite so that they don't eat as much. Unfortunately, most gyms are packed after 5 P.M. because so many people prefer to exercise at this time.

If you exercise at home after work, try to do so before dinner. But most importantly, do not exercise immediately before going to bed. Rather than exhausting you, exercise may actually invigorate you, making sleep difficult.

Men and Lifestyle

It is often believed that men live riskier lives than women. This idea could stem from men working in more danger-prone occupations such as a firefighter or police officer, but the fact is that men simply tend to engage in more dangerous lifestyle activities than women do.

Men are by nature aggressive creatures. It's part of their genetic and chemical makeup. In the past, aggression was necessary for survival. But today, rather than fighting saber-toothed tigers, many men engage in other high-adrenaline pursuits such as driving fast, drinking hard, or participating in extreme sports such as rock climbing and skydiving. In the eyes of many, living hard and fast is what defines masculinity; you're not a man unless you put your life on the line in some way on a regular basis.

Unfortunately, this mentality tends to reduce longevity by quite a few years. Hard drinkers risk a variety of medical problems, including liver disease and diabetes. Fast drivers risk serious physical injury or worse should they wreck—even if they're wearing seat belts. Participants of extreme sports wager they have at least one life left every time they engage in their favorite activity.

We're not going to tell you not to do any of these things, because that's not our place. The lifestyle choices you make are your own, and as such, you must live with the consequences. All we ask is that you take a moment to evaluate your lifestyle and see what you can do to make it even just a little bit healthier and safer. Extreme sports, for example, can be an incredible adrenaline rush, which is why most people engage in them. However, you should always take a moment to make sure your safety equipment is in good working order; it takes just one error in judgment to land you in the hospital or the morgue.

The same goes for any other potentially hazardous activity. If you think safety first and avoid unnecessary risks, you'll live a lot longer. This doesn't make you any less macho; it's just basic common sense.

Anti-aging and Women

When it comes to longevity, women have a decided advantage over men—despite the many physical changes they will undergo over their lifetime. On average, women live about seven and a half years longer than men and hold this advantage in life expectancy throughout the life cycle. The U.S. Census Bureau projects that the decided difference in life expectancy between men and women will continue to grow wider until around 2050, when the rates will begin to level off. At that point, say researchers, women can expect to live eighty-one years on average, and men can expect an average life expectancy of 71.8 years.

FACTS

Nature has gifted women with greater longevity than men, and that continues today despite recent advances in anti-aging medicine. In 1900, women lived an average of 51.5 years, compared to just 48.3 years for men. By 1950, women were living an average of 71.7 years compared to the male average of 66 years, and by 1990 women could expect to live 79 years compared to 72.1 years for men. What do women have that men don't? One answer is the hormone estrogen, which protects women from heart disease and stroke up until menopause, at which time estrogen levels subside and women's risk of heart disease equals that of men.

The reasons why women tend to live longer than men has been a topic of debate among health experts for years. Some speculate that women are just hardier creatures; others believe the difference is due to the fact that men, on average, are exposed to more environmental hazards than women. Let's take a quick look at some of the most current hypotheses on the issue.

- *Sex-linked differences.* One school of thought suggests that women at all ages have stronger immune resistance and are additionally protected from certain health problems by female hormones such as estrogen.
- *Exposure to environmental hazards.* In general, traditionally male occupations expose men to greater danger as well as more health and environmental hazards such as carcinogens. For example, health officials estimate that nearly 4 million workers—the majority of them men—have been or are currently exposed to asbestos and that approximately one-tenth of male lung cancer deaths are linked to asbestos exposure.
- *Differences in health habits.* Women, in general, tend to take better care of their health and avoid potentially harmful habits such as cigarette smoking and excessive alcohol consumption. This isn't to say, however, that smoking is no longer a health issue among women. Recent studies by the U.S. Department of Health and Human Services

have shown that smoking rates are gradually increasing among young women despite health warnings and education efforts.

- *Personality differences.* Far more men than women exhibit traits of the Type A personality—that is, more men than women tend to be hard driven, competitive, and extremely stressed. Unfortunately, while Type A individuals often make great corporate executives, their personalities also place them at much greater risk of heart disease, stroke, and a wealth of other health problems.

- *Differences in reaction to illness and disability.* When women start to get sick, they tend to seek immediate help. Men, on the other hand, tend to procrastinate until the condition can no longer be tolerated. This difference in reaction places men at greater risk of serious illness and, over the years, can adversely influence longevity.

Despite the natural protection that many women experience due to their gender, there are still many health issues with which they must contend and important steps they must take to ensure that they remain strong and healthy well into their later years.

Nutrition for Women

Women have unique nutritional needs with higher requirements than men of certain essential nutrients. However, many women tend to forget about or ignore their special dietary requirements and, in so doing, place their health in jeopardy and adversely affect their potential longevity. We'll review some of the most important nutrients for women.

Calcium

We touched on this earlier, but it bears repeating: Women need higher amounts of calcium than men because their physiology places them at greater risk of osteoporosis, or brittle bones, later in life. How important is this issue? Consider: Osteoporosis afflicts an estimated 25 million Americans, more than 80 percent of them women. The reason is simple: Women's bones are usually less dense to start with, and the reduction in estrogen that typically accompanies menopause can cause women to lose bone mass much more quickly. In addition, many women engage in calcium-inhibiting behaviors such as smoking, lack of weight-bearing exercise, and poor nutrition.

FACTS

In 1998, women accounted for 58 percent of those older than sixty-five and 70 percent of those eighty-five and older.

Ideally, women should begin consuming as many calcium-rich foods, such as milk and hard cheese, as early in life as possible. Bones grow more rapidly throughout childhood, adolescence, and young adulthood, so it's a good idea to get into the calcium habit at the onset of puberty and maintain it throughout your life. Women in their thirties should make extra sure they are getting sufficient calcium because bone mass begins to diminish after age thirty-five.

Calcium consumption is particularly important as women approach the age of menopause. Once the change of life hits, estrogen levels drop precipitously, and loss of bone mass begins with a vengeance. Those who have maintained strong, healthy bones throughout their lives will feel the effects far less than those who consumed minimal calcium.

The recommended daily allowance (RDA) of calcium for women over eighteen is 800 milligrams. However, some experts believe that isn't enough and recommend 1,000 milligrams daily for premenopausal women and 1,500 milligrams daily for postmenopausal women (and men over age sixty-five).

A woman's calcium needs also increase when she becomes pregnant, because the growing fetus leaches calcium from its mother. Government health officials recommend women take an additional 400 milligrams of the mineral during pregnancy and breastfeeding to compensate for what they lose. However, pregnant and breastfeeding women should avoid taking megadoses of calcium because it can pass into the breast milk.

Iron

Iron is an essential mineral necessary for the manufacture of hemoglobin, the red part of blood cells that carries oxygen throughout the body. Hemoglobin stores up to 70 percent of the body's iron supply, and additional iron is stored in muscle tissue to help deliver the oxygen needed to make the muscles contract.

Iron is important to both men and women, but women need higher levels of iron than men because they lose blood each month during their menstrual periods. The amount of blood lost typically isn't a lot, just a few spoonfuls for the average women. But if iron levels are already low, a heavy period can eventually lead to anemia, an inability of the blood to carry enough oxygen to the body's cells. Common symptoms of anemia include weakness, fatigue, irritability, headache, and recurring dizziness.

Most women receive sufficient levels of iron in their diet, particularly if they eat a lot of green leafy vegetables, which are a wonderful dietary source. However, women whose fast-paced lifestyle forces them into a steady diet of nutritionally poor fast food may find themselves iron deficient and headed toward a number of related health problems. The answer is better nutrition through a more varied and natural diet, or a daily iron supplement.

The RDA for iron is 18 milligrams for women up to age fifty and 10 milligrams for women fifty-one and older. (Older women need less iron because they cease to menstruate following menopause.) Women also need an additional 30 to 60 milligrams of iron daily during pregnancy and while breastfeeding, according to doctors. However, pregnant woman should not take iron supplements during their first trimester unless told to do so by their doctors. Megadoses of iron should also be avoided because of the possibility of iron toxicity.

You may notice that your stool turns black or gray after you start taking an iron supplement; this is normal and nothing to worry about. However, see your doctor immediately if you notice blood in your stool. It could mean you're taking too much.

Zinc

As noted earlier, zinc plays an important role in a variety of body functions and is essential for general health. It is required in trace amount, but many women are deficient nonetheless and should take steps to increase their zinc intake through dietary sources or a regular supplement. This is especially true for pregnant women, because zinc is vital to proper fetal growth and development.

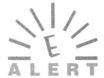

ALERT

Once a man passes the age of twenty-four, it is likely to take him longer to make his partner pregnant—regardless of his partner's age, report researchers in the journal *Human Reproduction*. Fecundity—the likelihood of achieving pregnancy within a certain period of time—is important because as the female ages, her ability to conceive declines dramatically, explains British fertility expert Dr. Christopher Barratt. If the man is not fecund, by the time he can impregnate his partner, it may too late because she is too old.

The RDA for zinc is 15 milligrams for all adults. Women should strive for an additional 5 milligrams daily when pregnant, and an extra 10 milligrams daily while breastfeeding. Too much zinc in sustained megadoses can result in zinc toxicity. Symptoms include nausea, vomiting, diarrhea, drowsiness, sluggishness, and light-headedness.

Women and Anti-aging Supplementation

The vast majority of anti-aging technologies and techniques can be safely used by both men and women of all ages. There are, however, one or two that are aimed specifically at men and that should be avoided by women due to the risk of potential side effects.

The most obvious, of course, is testosterone. The so-called "male sex hormone," testosterone is responsible for the sex drive in both men and women, though it plays a far more important role in the overall health of men. A testosterone deficiency in men can accelerate the aging process. In fact, researchers have had great success in reversing many of the common symptoms of aging by dosing older men with testosterone supplements.

Some researchers have also had good success using small amounts of testosterone to ease the symptoms of menopause in hormone-sensitive women undergoing hormone replacement therapy. But, in general, testosterone supplementation poses too many potential side effects to be of much use to women regardless of their age. Potential problems include masculinization (unwanted body hair and a deepening of the voice), oily skin, acne, elevated blood pressure, and an increased risk of heart disease.

On the flip side, men cannot enjoy the benefits of the female sex hormone estrogen, which is produced naturally up to menopause and available in prescription form following menopause. The health and age-reducing benefits of estrogen are many, including protection from heart disease, stroke, osteoporosis, and other potentially serious health problems.

One last warning: Certain man made and herbal dietary supplements should be used with caution if at all by women who are pregnant or postmenopausal. For example, high doses of retinol-type vitamin A can be harmful if taken during pregnancy. And ginseng has a mild estrogenic effect that can cause vaginal bleeding in postmenopausal women—a situation that can easily be mistaken as a symptom of uterine cancer. To avoid potential problems, make sure your doctor okays all dietary supplements while you are pregnant and is aware of any supplements you may be taking if you are postmenopausal.

Pregnancy and Child Rearing: How It Can Affect Your Aging

With the possible exception of menopause, few events in a woman's life affect her physical and mental well-being like pregnancy. How a woman handles the many demands of childbearing can play an important role in both her own long-term health and longevity and that of her unborn baby.

When a woman becomes pregnant, everything she does takes on greater importance, from the foods she eats, to her exercise regimen, to her personal lifestyle. A woman who approaches pregnancy well informed and willing to make the necessary changes her condition requires can expect to give birth to a healthy baby, as well as maintain her own good health. However, women with little social support, who are medically ignorant, or who refuse to give up bad habits place not only themselves but also their babies at risk. And in so doing, they are probably knocking years off of both of their lives.

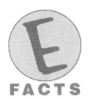

FACTS

Women experience sleep problems much more often than men, due in part to physiological changes as a result of menstruation, pregnancy, childbirth, breastfeeding, and menopause.

Starting Your Children Off Right

Staying young and healthy should be a lifelong goal, not something to be started only in middle age or our senior years. While many benefits can come from instituting a more healthful lifestyle after age forty, studies show that the greatest effects are derived when healthful living is a habit started early in life.

And just as we're never too old to start thinking young, neither are we ever too young. In fact, the greatest gift we can give our children is good health and an early start toward improved longevity.

Unfortunately, many people begin at an early age the bad habits that will plague them throughout their lives, habits that may have a detrimental impact on how well they will age and how long they will live. Children today, mesmerized by television, video games, and the Internet, live a more sedentary lifestyle than ever before. They don't eat properly, and they rarely exercise as much as they should. Worse, as more and more physical education programs fall by the wayside, the victims of budget cuts, we can't even count on our schools to keep our young people active. That means parents must take up the slack when it comes to ensuring that their children live with health in mind. They must make sure that their children eat right (at least at home) and that they get at least some exercise, even if it's just yard work. The importance of this can't be overstated. We're experiencing an epidemic of juvenile obesity, and the majority of overweight kids grow up to be overweight adults. Those extra pounds will impact on their health every day of their lives, increasing their risk of chronic illness and reducing the number of healthful years they can expect to live.

Here are a few stats for you to mull over, courtesy of the American Heart Association:

- More than 50 percent of children exceed the recommended intake of fat and cholesterol (a major contributor: greasy fast food).
- Children who overeat foods that are high in saturated fat tend to have higher cholesterol levels, which contributes to arteriosclerosis.
- Children who eat a lot of salty foods and are overweight are more likely to have high blood pressure.

As you can see, it's vitally important that parents take an active role in their children's nutrition and overall health. For many parents, this means making sure their children get all their vaccinations every year. This is important, to be sure, but there's much more to it than that. As young people mature, it becomes increasingly difficult to monitor their activities and make sure they do the right thing when it comes to their health. But while we can't be with them all the time, we can instill in them at a very early age the importance of taking care of their bodies through proper nutrition, adequate exercise, and avoiding harmful habits such as cigarette smoking, alcohol consumption, and drug use. All of this will go a long way toward helping future generations stay healthy throughout their lives and making sure those lives are as long as possible.

Here are a few quick tips to help you ensure your child's long-term health:

- Talk to your child about nutrition and health during the child's early years. Explain in a playful way the benefits of healthful foods and the potential hazards of junk foods.
- Make physical activity fun rather than a chore. If possible, exercise with your child; both of you will benefit.
- Encourage your child to participate in extracurricular sports.
- The American Heart Association recommends that parents limit fat intake for healthy children aged two years and older to 30 percent of their daily calories and that they consume no more than 300 milligrams of cholesterol per day. The American Academy of Pediatrics puts the recommended percentage of fat between 30 and 40 percent.
- The American Academy of Pediatrics and the National Heart, Lung, and Blood Institute suggest that children with a family history of heart disease have their blood cholesterol levels tested. Many

pediatricians recommend screening even when a child is not thought to be at high risk. Screening may reveal a potential problem that can be traced back to a parent who was unaware of the presence of a cardiovascular risk.

- Discuss with your child the potential harm of smoking. If you're a smoker yourself, make the effort to quit. Studies show that many lifelong smokers come from families that smoked and that many young people receive their first cigarette from an older family member or friend.

- Make yourself readily available should your child have any questions about his or her health or the many peer problems he or she is likely to face outside the home. Open communication can go a long way in helping children avoid a health crisis.

You can't be by your child's side every moment of his or her life, but you can help make your child aware early on of what's good and what's bad when it comes to his or her health. In doing so, you're also beginning an important anti-aging regimen that could add decades to your child's life span.

Anti-aging and Children

We've touched on the issue of anti-aging and children only briefly in this book because the vast majority of age-slowing technologies and techniques are designed for adults. It would be unsafe and extremely inappropriate for anyone under eighteen to sample today's most popular anti-aging agents, such as human growth hormone, DHEA, or testosterone, and no reputable physician would participate in such an endeavor.

But that doesn't mean young people can't begin an anti-aging regimen. It's never too early to start thinking with longevity in mind, and many of the practices and habits developed in one's early years can be of great benefit in the decades to come.

The most important thing young people can do to add years to their lives is maintain a healthful lifestyle that includes a proper diet, regular exercise, avoiding unhealthy habits such as tobacco and illicit drugs, and constantly monitoring the safety of their environment. I know I'm starting to sound like a broken record on these issues, but they're an extremely important aspect of any anti-aging approach, and even more so for children.

Diet

Most young people consume two separate diets—the food they receive at home, and the food they obtain on their own. Not surprisingly, most of the food purchased by young people today is of the junk or fast food variety—that is, hamburgers, hot dogs, french fries, soft drinks, and milk shakes. The occasional fast-food hamburger is okay, but a regular diet of greasy, fried foods poses a serious nutritional threat with long-term consequences that include obesity and related disorders.

As a result, it's the parents' responsibility to make sure that their children are eating right. This means providing plenty of fresh fruits and vegetables, fish, poultry, pasta, legumes, whole grain foods, and milk and other dairy products and minimal amounts of red meat and fried, fatty foods. Creating healthful meals every day can be a challenge for today's on-the-go families, but it's worth the effort when it comes to your child's current and future health.

Children go through different food phases as they grow up. During their toddler years, they often fixate on certain foods and may eat nothing else for days. Or they may demand seconds of a particular food one day and refuse to eat it the next. This is normal behavior and nothing to worry about. A four-day diet of grilled cheese sandwiches will do a child no harm, particularly if he or she supplements it with more healthful items such as carrot sticks or other sliced veggies. Even though a picky eater may fixate on a particular food at lunch or dinner, chances are good that he or she is actually eating a wide assortment of foods throughout the day.

The key to success is providing a broad range of foods for your children and explaining to them at an early age why proper nutrition is so important to their health. By doing this, you're helping to ensure that they eat right throughout their lives.

As for the food your children buy on their own, well, there's little you can do about that except try to counter it with healthful meals at home.

Young people like to snack, and fast food often provides an opportunity for them to socialize with friends and classmates. As long as your children don't make fast food a three-meal-a-day habit, they should be fine.

According to nutrition experts, adolescents and teenagers should consume the following food daily:

- *Four servings of milk and dairy products.* This can include low-fat milk, low-fat cheese, cottage cheese, and yogurt. Ice cream, while technically a dairy product, generally contains too much sugar and fat to be considered a nutritious alternative.
- *Three or more servings of fruit.* This can include fresh fruit, canned fruit, or fruit juice.
- *Three or more servings of vegetables, plus two or more servings of vegetables rich in vitamin A.* They can be cooked or raw.
- *Six to 8 ounces of meats, fish, poultry, and legumes.* Most servings are between 2 and 6 ounces. Make sure meat and poultry are lean.
- *Four or more servings of breads, cereals, and starchy vegetables.* This can include two slices of whole grain or enriched bread, a large bagel or muffin, 1 cup of dry cereal, or 1 cup of cooked cereal, pasta, or rice.

In addition, it makes sense for children to take a daily multivitamin tablet, just to make sure they're receiving the recommended daily allowance of vitamins, minerals, and other nutrients.

Exercise

Recent government and university studies have concluded that more young people are obese today than at any other time in American history. Over the past twenty years, researchers say, obesity in children aged six to eleven years has increased by 54 percent, and in teens, the increase is a frightening 39 percent. Twice as many young people now fall into the "super obese" category, which means they weigh at least 40 percent more than they should.

Reasons include poor dietary habits, a more sedentary lifestyle (thanks to video games and computers), and, perhaps most importantly, a lack of exercise. Sadly, obese youngsters generally grow up to become obese adults and, consequently, suffer from all of the related health problems. Worse, they are more likely to be viewed with ridicule and disapproval by classmates, teachers, and others, resulting in poor self-esteem and learning difficulties.

Young people benefit from exercise just as much as adults, but getting young people to exercise regularly can be a challenge. One way to instill the importance of exercise in your children is to be a role model. When you exercise, ask your children if they would like to accompany you. This benefits them physically and mentally and also provides an opportunity for you to bond.

Extracurricular sports, whether through school or an outside organization, are another way for young people to get the exercise they need. Football, baseball, swimming, track, tennis, soccer, cheerleading, and other activities go a long way toward helping young people stay physically fit and psychologically motivated. Children who express an interest in extracurricular sports should be encouraged to participate in them, but never force a child to participate in a sport if he or she doesn't want to. Forcing a child to play a sport will generate antagonism, anger, and poor performance, and the healthful aspects of the sport will be lost.

At the very least, don't let your children spend all of their free time surfing the Net, watching TV, or playing video games. Make sure at least some of their chores involve outdoor activities, such as yard work, and praise them when they take the exercise initiative.

Lifestyle

Childhood is a time of experimentation and pushing boundaries, of developing a sense of self as well as a sense of community with friends and peers. What often makes little sense to parents makes perfect sense to young people who are slowly, tentatively making their way into the world.

It's during adolescence and young adulthood that most of us develop a sense of lifestyle. Very often this mimics the environment in which we were raised, though sometimes it may take a completely different and unexpected turn. Much thought should go into our sense of lifestyle because it can have a dramatic impact on our current and future health.

Parents can guide their children's sense of lifestyle through example and gentle encouragement, and this can go a long way toward ensuring a healthful future. But the opposite is true, too. If you smoke, there's a better chance your children will smoke, regardless of how often you tell them, "Do as I say, not as I do." The same goes for other things such as alcohol consumption, exercise, and basic safety concerns such as the use of seat belts. The media can lecture young people on these issues all day long, but it still won't have as much impact as parental example.

Peer pressure is another important factor. Young people who hang around with peers who smoke are more likely to smoke themselves. The same goes for drug use and sexual experimentation, both of which can have tremendous long-term health consequences. You can't choose your children's friends, but you can guide them down a strong, healthful, moral path and educate them starting at an early age about what's right and what's not.

Anti-aging and the Senior Population

It's not uncommon for older people to believe that the anti-aging revolution has passed them by. Youth is for the young, they reason, and it's pointless to try to boost longevity when you're already in your sixties, seventies, or older.

How wrong they are! The truth is that there are two distinct perspectives to the anti-aging mind-set. The first is that the battle against aging begins in early youth and involves living a healthful life and taking advantage of anti-aging technologies and techniques where safe and appropriate. The goal is not only to increase our life span but also to ensure that our later years are healthy and vital.

The second perspective is that you're never too old to be young, or, more colloquially, you're only as old as you feel. This is a very healthy attitude toward aging because it focuses on the positive aspects of one's senior years rather than the negatives, which is contrary to what our society tends to do. It also places responsibility for slowing the aging process on the individual and forces him or her to take an active role in anti-aging and overall health maintenance.

Anti-aging Technologies and the Elderly

Many of the most popular and promising approaches to slowing the aging process, such as human growth hormone, DHEA, and testosterone supplementation, appear to be perfect for those sixty-five years and older. These techniques replace important hormones and other substances known or believed to diminish over the years and, thus, help slow or reverse the aging processing by revitalizing the mind and body. Many men who have received testosterone or DHEA report renewed vigor, physical strength, stamina, libido, and mental clarity—a sure sign that these compounds will play an important role in the anti-aging revolution.

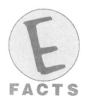

FACTS

Until very recently, doctors were convinced that testosterone was more of an enemy than a friend to men. The hormone, they believed, was one of the major contributors to early-life heart disease, and it caused men to die younger than women. However, several new studies suggest that testosterone may not be the death dealer we thought it was. All of this is good news for older men considering testosterone supplements to help prevent some of the more common age-related problems, such as osteoporosis (which afflicts men as well as women), poor muscle tone, decreased libido, and depression.

However, as promising as these technologies are, they should be approached with caution. Some still require quite a bit of additional research regarding safety and efficacy before the mainstream scientific community will offer its stamp of approval, and others, while generally acknowledged as effective, come with warnings and caveats. DHEA, for example, can lead to liver damage if taken in high quantities. And because the compound is a precursor for estrogen and testosterone, it's possible that DHEA could encourage the growth of tumors stimulated by these hormones (i.e., tumors of the breast, uterus, or prostate).

Human growth hormone is another promising anti-aging compound that should be viewed cautiously by older people. In one six-month study of healthy men over age sixty, recipients of human growth hormone experienced an increase in muscle mass and skin thickness, a decrease in total body fat, and a slight boost in calcium levels in the lower spine. However, a twelve-month follow-up study found that many of these youthful benefits had started to reverse. And another study found that while there were noticeable increases in muscle tissue and a decrease in fat, there were no significant improvements in muscle strength, endurance, or functional ability, nor were there improvements in mental function. Many test subjects also experienced various side effects that necessitated a reduction in dose.

It's interesting to note that some studies have found that another chemical, known as insulin-like growth factor, appears to be the real cause of many of the benefits associated with human growth hormone. The compounds work closely together, and some scientists speculate that one day, insulin-like growth factor will replace human growth hormone as a better, more effective weapon in the war on aging.

In addition to the possibility of side effects and less than impressive results, many of today's most promising anti-aging compounds and technologies are available by prescription only, are extremely expensive, and only very rarely covered by insurance, which puts them out of the reach of many older Americans.

Adhering Your Lifestyle to Your Age

Because many anti-aging techniques and technologies are experimental and still being studied, they may be inappropriate for a large percentage of America's seniors. But if you're still intrigued and feel you would benefit from something like testosterone or DHEA, talk with your doctor and follow his or her advice.

Of course, the latest scientific advances aren't the only way to slow the progress of Father Time. A growing number of today's over-sixty set are finding that living a healthful lifestyle can be just as effective and a lot less expensive or risky. This means eating with nutrition in mind, exercising as much as you're able, and maintaining strong social support.

Diet

A frightening percentage of older Americans eat so poorly that it affects their health. Many are forced into this cycle by a fixed income or other financial factors; others eat primarily fast food or microwavable processed meals because they live alone and find it more convenient.

We've dealt with the importance of nutrition throughout this book, but the elderly are at particular risk. Following are some simple dietary suggestions for better health and longevity:

- *Eat more fruits, vegetables, and grains.* These foods provide much-needed complex carbohydrates and plenty of fiber, which can keep you "regular," lower your cholesterol level, and help prevent certain types of cancer. Fresh fruits and vegetables are also important sources of vital nutrients, including age-fighting antioxidants. Try to eat five or more servings every day.
- *Reduce your intake of fat and cholesterol.* This will go a long way toward reducing your risk of heart disease, stroke, certain types of cancer, and other medical problems. Doctors recommend following this advice as early in life as possible, but it's never too late to start. If your diet consists of red meat five nights a week, try substituting pasta, dinner-size salads, and fish.
- *Eat more low-fat protein.* The need for protein increases slightly as we age, yet many older people tend to eat less than they did when they were younger. In the minds of many, protein means red meat, but as you get older, it's important that you get your protein with as little fat as possible. How? By increasing your consumption of legumes, nuts, and grains. They can be eaten in a wide variety of ways, and they're far less expensive than meat.
- *Watch your salt.* A common complaint among older people is a reduction in their senses of taste and smell, which in turn results in the need for more salt and other spices in the foods they eat. However, sensitivity to salt increases with age, which means additional risk for people with age-related health problems such as hypertension, heart disease, and kidney disease. People who are in good health

have less to worry about from salt, but it's still wise to keep your salt intake to a minimum. If your food tastes bland, try a salt-free seasoning substitute.

- *Reduce your caffeine and alcohol intake.* Sensitivity to both chemicals increases as people age, so we feel their effects much more than when we were younger. Neither caffeine nor alcohol does us much good, so it's wise to cut down—if you can't eliminate them altogether.

- *Drink more water.* Dehydration is a common problem among the elderly, especially those who live alone. The solution is simple: Drink as much water as you can, all day long. At a minimum, you should consume eight glasses of plain water a day, and more if possible. Just keep a sports bottle with you wherever you go and refill it as necessary. And coffee, beer, and soft drinks don't count as water!

Anti-aging and the Differently Abled

The differently abled are often left out when it comes to anti-aging research, but there's no reason why those with chronic conditions or physical impairments can't take advantage of current technologies and techniques, as long as they are medically appropriate and do not interfere with required therapies or medications.

The truth is that the differently abled really aren't all that different. They may face certain limitations as a result of their health or disability, but as long as they live a relatively healthful lifestyle and are in good general health, they should benefit from today's most popular anti-aging approaches just as well as anyone else.

However, before taking over-the-counter anti-aging supplements or engaging in any other dramatic lifestyle or dietary changes, it's a good idea to consult with your physician if you have a chronic health condition or disability that could be affected by such changes. Certain foods can react adversely with certain medications, and some anti-aging supplements may result in physical changes that could affect medical treatment. Even though the majority of over-the-counter supplements are considered generally safe and effective, it's always wise to get your doctor's okay first.

It's important to note that many simple anti-aging lifestyle changes may also benefit those with chronic conditions or physical disabilities. Regular exercise, for example, can improve overall physical and mental health and can even complement ongoing physical therapy. And there's no downside to improved nutrition. Eating right helps strengthen the mind and body, improves stamina, and boosts the immune system. Regardless of physical limitations, exercise and diet are two of the most powerful weapons we have when it comes to winning the war against aging.

CHAPTER 10
Stay Informed

It is always important to be as informed as possible, especially when it comes to an aspect of your life such as aging. If you are serious about your anti-aging regimen, you will want to pay close attention to this chapter and work to stay abreast of the latest theories and findings. In this chapter, we are going to examine anti-aging research through the ages, with a special emphasis on the most recent breakthroughs and the field's bright future.

Anti-aging Research

Our quest to slow the aging process is far from a modern phenomenon. In fact, nearly every ancient culture, from the Egyptians to the Chinese, has put forth its own theories and principles on why we age and what can be done to slow it down. Some were based on science or philosophy, others in myth and legend. But the goal for all was the same—perpetual youth.

The centuries have witnessed a greater understanding of the physiology of human aging but very little in ways to slow it down. Almost every era has had its share of potions, pills, and elixirs "guaranteed" to keep users forever young, but all have turned out to be ineffective placebos, at best, or dangerous concoctions of toxic chemicals, at worst.

Today, there is growing talk of an all-in-one supplement of youth-preserving nutrients, enzymes, and other compounds that will keep old age at bay, but such a pill is undoubtedly still many, many years away. Nonetheless, the secret of slow aging, if not perpetual youth, has never been closer at hand. Every day, medical researchers discover new and better compounds that promise to keep every part of the human machine running at full capacity, with minimal wear and tear. This is great news not only for babies who are born today but also for men and women who were born fifty years ago. Old age still can't be stopped (in fact, it may never be), but it can be controlled with greater success than ever before.

Successful Aging

Before discussing anti-aging research, it's important that we define the concept of successful aging. This is a very subjective issue, and no doubt everyone has a slightly different definition, though most people would probably agree with "living to a ripe old age in relatively good physical health."

However, most gerontologists would say this is only a partial definition at best. As we learned earlier, there are many other components to the aging process besides physical health, and they all have an equal place in the definition of successful aging.

Take, for example, the psychological and emotional aspects of growing older. Could you define the aging process as successful if you were in perfect physical condition but incapacitated by anxiety or depression? Certainly not. How about being physically fit but an emotional mess? Again, the answer would have to be no.

When discussing anti-aging research, the definition of success must incorporate all aspects of the aging process. Living 150 years would be a fool's goal if we were tormented by side effects from the technologies that made extreme longevity a reality, or if we lacked the social support of family and friends, or if our bodies stayed young but our minds did not.

All of these factors have an individual role, but it is clear that they also strongly affect each other. If we're physically frail or in chronic pain, happiness probably will not be our primary emotion, nor will we be at our psychological best. Similarly, a distressed emotional or psychological state will almost certainly take a heavy toll on our physical well-being. These components are interlocking parts of the human machine; when one starts to go, all are affected.

Ultimately, the simplest and most accurate definition of successful aging is "living as long as we want to live in a sound physical, psychological, and emotional condition." To extend life without considering the impact of greater longevity on our quality of life is medical meddling that borders on cruelty.

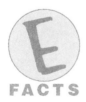

FACTS

All human cells contain genes that cause them to self-destruct if they become damaged or infected, or as part of the regulation of cell numbers during normal development. This "cellular suicide" is known as apoptosis, and it plays an integral role in life. Examples of apoptosis at work include the following:

- The formation of the fingers and toes of the fetus by removing the tissue between them.
- The elimination of surplus cells in the brain to guarantee the proper formation of connections between neurons.
- The elimination of cells irrevocably infected by viruses or with damaged DNA.

Anti-aging Research Through History

Man has approached the mystery of aging from a wide variety of directions. Over the centuries and through many diverse cultures, advancing age has been blamed on everything from angry gods to an imbalance in the body's humors. Techniques to slow down the aging process have been equally bizarre (by contemporary standards) and almost universally unsuccessful.

The ancient Greeks were some of the first to tackle aging from both a medical and a philosophical perspective, concluding that age had much to do with the body's four essential "humors"—blood, phlegm, yellow bile, and black bile.

According to the Greek philosopher Empedocles (c. 490–430 B.C.), nature is made up of four root elements—earth, wind, fire, and water; these very different elements combined in varying proportions to create all living creatures, from plants on up. If one accepted that theory, then it made sense that illness, infirmity, and all of the common signs of advancing age were caused by an imbalance in the body's four humors. Empedocles also speculated that nature was influenced by two different and opposing forces, which he called love and strife. Love, he noted, binds things together; strife separates them. Therefore, if you have too much strife in your life, you will age. Interestingly, modern anti-aging researchers incorporated Empedocles' concept of opposing forces into the theory of cellular disorder, or entropy.

Other ancient theories on aging and ways to slow it were equally innocent and amusing (again, by contemporary standards), as were attempts to hold age in check. Over the years, so-called wizards, alchemists, and con artists of every stripe took full advantage of man's quest for eternal youth, selling worthless pills and potions to a gullible public desperate to hold on to its fleeting youth.

It wasn't until the nineteenth century that science started to enter the picture. A French physiologist named Charles-Edouard Brown-Sequard made a name for himself late in the century by promoting the anti-aging benefits of extracts derived from crushed animal testicles. Subsequent studies ultimately proved Brown-Sequard wrong, though he must be given some credit for advancing the theory that hormonal-endocrine agents may play a role in slowing the aging process—a concept contemporary researchers are studying with high hopes.

It wasn't until the 1940s that medical researchers really began to put forth hard science theories on why the body ages. One of the most popularly received theories was that of genetic mutation, which speculated that increasing mistakes at the chromosomal level result in physical deterioration and, thus, the most common signs of advancing age, such as wrinkles and graying hair.

This theory gained still greater acceptance in the early 1960s, when renowned anatomist Leonard Hayflick uncovered the primary principles of cellular aging, a finding that continues to have immense implications in anti-aging research. Hayflick proved beyond a doubt that cells have a very specific lifespan, dividing only a preprogrammed number of times, then stopping. He also noted during laboratory studies that cells from older people tend to die more quickly than cells from younger test subjects, a finding that supports the concept that the aging process could be slowed if only the body's "aging clock" could somehow be reset. The key, of course, remains in finding that special "clock." So far, researchers have been unsuccessful.

Anti-aging Research: The Latest Findings

Anti-aging research has become one of the hottest areas of medical science in recent years, as aging baby boomers have increasingly demanded safe and effective ways to maintain their diminishing youth. And the world's pharmaceutical companies and major medical research facilities are eager to comply, knowing full well the huge financial windfall that awaits the corporation that develops the first successful anti-aging pill or potion.

Of course, this Fountain of Youth is no doubt many years away. So much about the aging process remains a mystery that the chances of creating an actual anti-aging pill—a magic bullet that will stop aging in its tracks—will likely remain a pipe dream for decades to come.

But that doesn't mean we have to stand idly by while our skin wrinkles, our energy diminishes, and our hair turns gray. An eclectic array of medical approaches have shown success in slowing or reversing the effects of aging, some more so than others. Here are a few of the most promising.

The Antioxidant Approach

Antioxidants, as noted earlier, are substances that help prevent the cellular damage done by free radicals. Our body produces some antioxidants naturally, and we consume others in the food we eat. In fact, many fruits and vegetables are veritable antioxidant factories, rich with healthful compounds. Even though the association between free radicals and aging is still under investigation, several studies have confirmed that increasing the body's arsenal of antioxidants can, indeed, help diminish the ravages of age and protect us from age-related disease such as heart disease and certain forms of cancer.

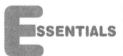 **ESSENTIALS**

Our bodies produce antioxidants naturally, but we also get these cell-saving compounds from the foods we eat. The best way to keep your body supercharged with antioxidants is to maintain a diet rich in fruits and vegetables—at least 2.5 cups a day, and preferably more. The best antioxidant sources include blueberries, cherries, pink grapefruit, oranges, prunes, raisins, red grapes, strawberries, alfalfa sprouts, broccoli sprouts, brussels sprouts, onions, red bell peppers, and spinach.

The first breakthrough in antioxidant research occurred in 1969, when researchers identified an important antioxidant known as superoxide dismutase (SOD), an enzyme that breaks down superoxide—one of the most powerful free radicals in the body. The link between aging and cellular damage caused by free radicals seemed strong, but researchers were unable to confirm it definitively. The question remained, Could life be extended by reducing oxidative damage?

Researchers at the University of Southern California wanted to find out, so they bred fruit flies with a special protein that could increase the activity of SOD and other antioxidants when the flies were exposed to heat. The specially engineered flies were raised side by side with a group of normal, equally aged fruit flies. When the insects were five days old, they were exposed to pulses of heat that were expected to increase free radical activity and stimulate their antioxidant defenses.

The researchers were stunned by the experiment's results. The normal fruit flies died long before their six-week lifespan, but those with more SOD lived almost 50 percent longer.

More recently, researchers at Southern Methodist University in Dallas, Texas, created another batch of fruit flies that were genetically altered to produce higher levels of SOD and another natural antioxidant known as catalase. Those flies also lived substantially longer than their nongenetically altered brethren and appeared to age more slowly. Key improvements included more energy, faster movements, and noticeably less damage from free radicals.

Of course, fruit flies and humans are much more different than they are the same, and similar studies will have to be performed on mammals before researchers can state authoritatively that boosting the body's natural antioxidant production reduces the effects of the aging process. But the concept looks promising, and nutrition experts are already touting a diet rich in antioxidants such as vitamins C and vitamin E as a way of reducing free radical damage, especially among smokers and other high-risk, fast-aging groups.

Another important area of research is determining exactly where free radicals perform the most harm and coming up with ways to stop it. The goal, say medical researchers at Ontario's University of Guelph and elsewhere, is to focus therapies on the most important injured cells rather than attacking free radicals scattershot throughout the entire body. Slowing the aging process is one goal of this research, but scientists also hope that it will allow them to help people with degenerative disorders such as familial amyotrophic lateral sclerosis. Individuals with this disease tend to die younger than normal; they also have heavily damaged motor neurons and mutations in SOD.

The results of these and similar experiments are all very promising, but researchers still don't know exactly why antioxidants help slow the aging process. When that mystery is finally solved, the life-extending potential could be explosive.

The Starvation Approach

Would you be willing to eliminate all of your favorite foods and reduce your caloric intake to almost starvation levels if it would help you live longer? Most people would probably say no, yet this technique—known scientifically as caloric restriction—has proved extremely successful at slowing the aging process in animals and exhibits similar promise in expanding the lifespan of humans as well.

The downside is that you're thin and almost constantly hungry and cold. For caloric restriction to have any kind of impact on longevity, practitioners must eat up to 50 percent less than they normally would. This means going from an average of 2,100 calories a day to just 1,500 calories, eating several smaller meals rather than three large ones, and consuming primarily fruits and vegetables.

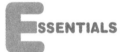
ESSENTIALS

Since 1986, Michael Cooper, a former electrical engineer currently studying biology at Southern Methodist University, has subsisted on a diet that most others would find far too limiting to maintain and has gradually reduced his daily caloric intake from 2,800 to 1,500. Over the years, his weight has dropped from 160 pounds to a very lean 120. Is it all worth it? Cooper admits that so far he hasn't seen much of a slowdown in the aging process. And he notes that because of his lean physique, he looks older than he actually is.

As unappetizing as this sounds, some people are actually living the lifestyle. And many researchers say caloric restriction could hold some very important clues to hyperlongevity.

The benefits of caloric restriction were first noted nearly sixty-five years ago by a Cornell University researcher named Clive M. McKay. He found that keeping rats slightly undernourished actually helped them live longer.

Numerous subsequent studies on laboratory animals proved beyond a doubt the effectiveness of caloric restriction. Animals placed on very restrictive diets exhibit an increase in both their average and maximum life spans, and the fewer calories they consume, the greater the increase. Mice placed on caloric restriction from a very early age live up to fifty-six months, compared to an average lifespan of thirty-nine months for mice who ate a normal calorie-rich diet. Nutritionally restricted animals also demonstrate a stronger immune system and have dramatically less incidence of age-related diseases, including heart disease, cancer, cataracts, and kidney disease. This suggests that in humans, extreme caloric restriction can prevent these ailments as well as the development of debilitating degenerative disorders such as Alzheimer's disease and Parkinson's disease.

Caloric restriction has been tested on a wide variety of species, ranging from insects to primates, with very similar results. The greatest benefits, however, were seen in those subjects that started the regimen from an early age and supplemented their restrictive diet with plenty of vitamins and minerals. It is important to understand that there's a huge difference between undernourished and malnourished.

But as with all promising anti-aging concepts, caloric restriction raises far more questions than it answers. Researchers know that undernourished animals live longer, but they don't know why. What is it about consuming fewer calories that extends longevity so dramatically? And while it has shown tremendous potential on laboratory animals, will it have a similar effect on human beings?

Medical researchers agree that the restrictive diet needed to extend longevity is far too harsh for most people to pursue. We're used to eating anything we want any time we want, and even greater longevity isn't prize enough for us to give that up. As a result, researchers are struggling to understand how caloric restriction works with the goal of developing a more acceptable alternative that provides the same beneficial effects.

While much about caloric restriction still remains a mystery, most researchers agree that the body's response to the diet is an evolutionary adaptation to periods of food scarcity. In short, when calories become less plentiful, the body goes into self-preservation mode, boosting internal defense mechanisms that increase lifespan. In the wild, the body returns to its normal state once food again becomes plentiful. But with an intentionally restrictive diet, the body is *always* in self-preservation mode.

Keep in mind that almost all research into caloric restriction has been conducted on laboratory animals. There are a number of people who have aggressively adapted the lifestyle in the hope of increasing their longevity, but it's far too soon to say for sure whether the diet works as well in people as it does in mice. That's something only time will tell.

The Natural Hormone Approach

Quite a bit of current anti-aging research centers around the rejuvenating effects of naturally occurring hormones, raising the question of whether aging is a result of diminishing levels of hormones or hormone deficiencies are a result of aging. Most steroid hormones are available only by prescription and for very specific uses, but word is spreading among anti-aging activists who see the tremendous potential they have in helping to slow the aging process.

Human Growth Hormone

One of the most promising compounds is human growth hormone (GH). This substance is released by the pituitary gland until around age thirty and is very important in our physical development. Levels of GH are highest when we're fetuses, decline during childhood, then increase again during adolescence. After age thirty, the production of GH slows considerably, and in many older people, it actually appears to cease completely.

The potential importance of GH in extending longevity is quite apparent, since it is clear that as levels of the hormone decline, so does body function. Clinical studies have shown a correlation between low levels of GH and a decline in muscle mass, an increase in body fat, reduced immune response, and other age-related conditions. So, the questions is, Could GH supplements help reduce these effects and, in effect, slow the aging process? A growing number of anti-aging specialists believe so.

In one of the most telling experiments, Dr. Daniel Rudman of the Medical College of Wisconsin and the Milwaukee VA Medical Center gathered twenty-one healthy men between the ages of sixty-one and eighty-one, all of whom had extremely low levels of growth hormone. Twelve of the men received injections of GH over a period of six months, and the remaining nine did not. The results? The men who received the GH supplements had a 14 percent reduction in body fat and a 9 percent increase in muscle mass. The men also said that the injections made them feel better than they had in years. However, the effects quickly wore off when the injections were stopped.

Subsequent studies confirmed the beneficial effects of human growth hormone. In addition to a reduction in body fat and an increase in muscle mass, many older people who have received GH injections also showed improved heart function, improved immune function, healthier cholesterol levels, more energy, improved sexual function, and other benefits.

Despite numerous studies proving the beneficial effects of GH on the aging process, the hormone is severely restricted in the United States; as of this writing, the only FDA approved use is for children with documented deficiencies. However, GH is widely available in other countries, and a growing number of anti-aging clinics are prescribing it to patients specifically to slow the effects of aging.

Caution on the part of the U.S. Food and Drug Administration is probably a good thing. Despite the good it does, studies show that growth hormone can result in serious side effects, including cancer, arthritis, and diabetes. It can also cause swelling and headaches even in low doses. Right now, the National Institutes of Health is funding several studies on GH to determine who, if anyone, would benefit from its use and what the optimum doses should be. As a result, it will be several years—if at all—before growth hormone becomes available to the general public in the United States.

Dehydroepiandrosterone (DHEA)

This steroid hormone, produced by the adrenal glands, is plentiful when we're young, though levels drop noticeably as we age. In fact, by age fifty, we produce less than a third of the amount of DHEA we produced when we were younger, and by age sixty, body levels of the hormone are almost undetectable.

DHEA is a very important hormone. It is used by the body to produce testosterone and estrogen. It also helps our immune systems stay strong and healthy.

Like human growth hormone, low levels of DHEA appear to promote the development of many health problems commonly associated with aging, including cancer and heart disease. In one clinical study of men between the ages of fifty and seventy-nine, researchers found that those with extremely low levels of DHEA had the highest rates of heart disease.

The health and longevity potential of DHEA is tremendous, say proponents. Several studies suggest that placing healthy individuals on a regimen of DHEA supplementation can reduce body fat, cut cholesterol levels, increase muscle mass, boost the immune system, and even ease depression. In women, DHEA has been shown to improve age-related osteoporosis by increasing formation of bone and increasing levels of estrogen and testosterone.

Animal studies have been equally impressive. In one remarkable experiment, DHEA supplements helped inhibit the growth of artificially planted tumors in elderly mice, and other studies suggest that the hormone can improve memory and even aid in weight reduction.

As the evidence builds, a growing number of physicians are placing their older patients on DHEA to reduce risk of disease, increase strength and vigor, and improve their chances of a long and healthy life. However, the hormone isn't for everyone, and there is the potential for serious side effects, researchers warn. Men with prostate cancer, pregnant women, or women with breast cancer or ovarian cancer should not take DHEA because the resulting hormone stimulation could actually worsen these conditions. Less serious side effects include liver irritation, hypertension, acne in men, and light facial hair in women, though these effects usually disappear when DHEA is stopped.

It's important to note that while the data regarding DHEA's efficacy in helping to slow the aging process continues to build, there have been no long-term human studies regarding its benefits.

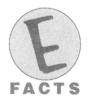

FACTS

Clinical studies have found that oral DHEA supplements can lower total serum cholesterol by an average of 18 percent without any changes in lifestyle.

Testosterone

Testosterone is often referred to as the male sex hormone. However, women also manufacture testosterone, albeit in much smaller levels—generally one-tenth the amount men do. Without it, neither gender would have much of a sex drive.

Testosterone is responsible for a large number of functions in men. In addition to promoting sexual desire and stimulating sperm production, it aids the growth of certain organs; promotes muscle, skin, and bone growth; nourishes the urinary and reproductive tissue; and stimulates prostate growth.

The effects of testosterone are most evident during puberty, during which time it plays an important role in the development of secondary sexual characteristics, including a deeper voice, body hair, increased muscle mass, and increased oil-gland secretions (a common cause of the teenage bane known as acne). Testosterone levels diminish gradually as men age, though production can be affected over time by a wide array of things, including illness, obesity, tobacco and alcohol use, lack of exercise, poor diet, and certain medications.

The body's levels of testosterone begin to diminish after puberty, with noticeable effects on physical health. However, several studies have found that testosterone supplementation later in life can help slow or reverse many of the problems associated with age-related testosterone deficiency, suggesting that the hormone could play an important role as a youth-preserving agent.

Several international studies, most of them involving men with noticeably low levels of testosterone due to old age or conditions such as hypogonadism, have demonstrated the hormone's amazing rejuvenating capabilities. In one eight-week study of twenty-nine subjects, almost all reported improved erectile function, libido, and mood, as well as increased energy. Another study involving men over fifty found that those who received testosterone supplements reported renewed strength, increased sex drive, and lower LDL cholesterol levels. And in a double-blind, placebo-controlled, crossover study, thirteen healthy elderly men with documented low testosterone levels were given 100 milligrams of testosterone weekly for three months.

Twelve members of the group reported significant behavior improvements, including feelings of well-being and increased libido.

In addition to improvements in mood and libido, several studies have found that testosterone supplements can help reduce the risk of heart disease and strengthen aging bones. This is an important finding because men with low testosterone levels are up to six times as likely to break their hip in a fall than men with normal hormone levels.

Prescription testosterone supplements via injection or transdermal patch can be a godsend to a lot of elderly men, but cautions and side effects must be considered. The biggest danger, say doctors, is the risk of worsening hormone-sensitive cancers such as prostate cancer. Testosterone can also influence HDL cholesterol levels and the risk of coronary heart disease.

Finally, the hormone should not be given to men who naturally maintain normal testosterone levels because of the risk of dangerous side effects and the possibility that oversupplementation can inhibit the body's normal testosterone production. To ensure that your body produces adequate levels of testosterone on its own, get plenty of exercise and consume a healthy diet. You'll be happy that you did in years to come.

Melatonin

Of all the hormones produced by your body, melatonin shows some of the greatest promise as an anti-aging wonder agent. First discovered in 1958, this compound—produced by the pineal gland—has demonstrated remarkable properties in everything from lifespan extension, to easing insomnia, to slowing cancer growth. And that's just the beginning, say researchers.

The pineal gland, which is located deep within the brain behind the eyes, is, in many ways, the body's clock. Stimulated by sunlight, it governs our circadian rhythms—the various processes that occur over a twenty-four-hour period, such as the sleep cycle. It also governs more long-term cycles such as a woman's monthly menstrual period. In addition, it is associated with various seasonal rhythms such as adapting to the shorter days of the fall and winter. Over our lifetime, the pineal gland orchestrates the release of key substances, including growth hormones, sexual hormones, and disease-fighting antibodies.

Some researchers believe that melatonin is the pineal gland's "messenger," that fluctuations in melatonin levels tell other body systems when to go to work, how hard to work, and when to slow down. Its responsibilities range from the onset of puberty to telling us when to go to sleep and when to wake up. Without melatonin, our lives would be a mess.

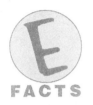

FACTS

According to researchers at the University of Texas, melatonin, a hormone produced by the pineal gland, is a very effective scavenger of cell-damaging free radicals.

The role of the pineal gland and melatonin in the aging process—and as a way of slowing down that process—is becoming increasingly clear as medical researchers gain greater understanding of the body's internal clock. Once we grow too old to reproduce (around the ages of forty-five to fifty for most women), the pineal gland begins to reduce production of melatonin, which in turn signals almost all other systems that it's time to "retire." Thus begins the aging process as we know it. Interestingly, women have a larger pineal gland than men, which could explain why women typically age more slowly and live longer.

Once we understand how the pineal gland and its vital messenger, melatonin, affect the body and help trigger the aging process, the potential role of the hormone in slowing that process becomes clearer. If we can maintain the level of melatonin we had at age thirty throughout our lives, will aging occur more slowly? In theory, the answer is yes. By tricking the pineal gland with melatonin supplements, we should remain biologically young while growing chronologically older.

Clinical studies on mice show great promise in this area. Dr. Walter Pierpaoli, an immunologist at the Biancalana-Masera Foundation for the Aged in Ancona, Italy, and Dr. Vladmir Lesnikov of the Institute of Experimental Medicine in St. Petersburg, Russia, cross-transplanted the pineal glands between the brains of old and young mice. The results? Young mice that received the pineal glands from older mice began to age much faster, while the older mice that received pineal glands from younger mice actually regained many characteristics of youth and stayed healthy throughout their lifespan.

The addition of melatonin also appears to stimulate the immune system, which usually weakens with age. Part of the reason for this weakening is the degeneration of the thymus, a tiny gland that plays a huge role in our ability to combat disease due to large concentrations of disease-fighting white blood cells known at T lymphocytes. The thymus more than doubles in size during puberty but degenerates by more than 90 percent by age sixty-five. The result is a diminished immune system.

Dr. Pierpaoli studied the influence of melatonin on reduced immune function by adding the hormone to the drinking water of elderly mice. The results were impressive. Almost all of the mice who received the hormone experienced a noticeable boost in their immune function. In addition, the weight of their thymus glands increased, and their thymus cells became much more active.

Studies have shown that melatonin has many other benefits as well. They include the following:

- *Slowing tumor growth.* Researchers at Tulane University School of Medicine report studies that suggest that melatonin can effectively inhibit the growth of human breast cancer cells. And in Milan, Italy, cancer specialists have started adding melatonin to chemotherapy and immunotherapy as a way of reducing the side effects of these cancer treatments. Extra benefits include additional tumor regression and greater patient longevity.
- *Improving quality of sleep.* Numerous studies have proved melatonin a safe and effective treatment for people with sleep difficulties. Best of all, there are no apparent side effects.
- *Easing jet lag.* Several studies involving overseas travelers have found that melatonin can help reset the body's natural clock, easing the effects of jet lag and inducing restful sleep.
- *Reducing risk of heart disease.* Melatonin has shown great efficacy in reducing blood cholesterol in patients with dangerously high levels.

Melatonin, which is available over the counter, appears safe when used in moderate doses (1 to 3 milligrams is common) and as recommended. However, researchers are quick to warn that there are no conclusive studies documenting the effects of long-term use. Erring on the side of caution, most doctors recommend that people under age forty-five (who naturally manufacture sufficient amounts of the hormone) refrain from using melatonin except for short-term use in the treatment of jet lag or insomnia. Those who should never use melatonin include pregnant or nursing women, women trying to become pregnant, people on prescription steroid medications, and individuals with autoimmune diseases such as multiple sclerosis and immune system cancers such as leukemia.

For best results, melatonin should be taken shortly before bedtime. Because of the risk of drowsiness, it's unwise to drive a car or operate heavy machinery after taking melatonin supplements.

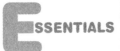
SSENTIALS

If proper nutrition, lots of exercise, and a healthy lifestyle doesn't give you immortality, you still have one last option—cryogenic preservation. It works like this: After you die, your body is pumped full of chemicals and frozen solid in liquid nitrogen until future scientists figure out a way to fix what killed you and then "reanimate" you. Of course, you have to wait awhile. But then, you have all the time in the world. Right now the whole concept is more science fiction than science fact. But to the men and women who have taken out special life insurance policies to pay for their cryogenic preservation when they finally die, it still beats the alternative.

The Mineral Approach

The importance of vitamins and minerals is drilled into our minds from a very early age, and millions of people now take a multivitamin tablet every day as part of their overall health regimen. These essential nutrients are instrumental in preventing disease and ensuring a strong mind and body—and some trace minerals, say medical researchers, may also help keep us young.

Chromium

One of the most promising of these compounds is chromium, a mineral that helps the body metabolize fat, convert blood sugar into energy, and make insulin work more efficiently. Chromium is derived primarily from our diet. Rich sources of this important nutrient include whole-grain foods, eggs, broccoli, orange juice, grape juice, seafood, dairy products, and many different types of meat. It is also available in supplement form, which is good for those who may be somewhat deficient due to poor dietary habits.

In addition to the benefits already noted, several recent studies have also shown that chromium plays the following important roles:

- *It protects the heart by lowering serum cholesterol levels and triglycerides.* In a study published in *The Western Journal of Medicine*, twenty-eight subjects with elevated cholesterol levels were given either 200 micrograms of chromium picolinate or a harmless placebo. By six weeks, those receiving the chromium picolinate saw a 7 percent decrease in total cholesterol, which reduced their risk of heart disease by 14 percent. Levels of low-density lipoprotein, the so-called "bad" cholesterol, dropped by more than 10 percent.
- *It prevents or aids in the management of diabetes by assisting in the production and metabolism of insulin.* To prove the effectiveness of chromium in controlling glucose (blood sugar), researchers with the U.S. Department of Agriculture divided rats into two groups—those on a chromium-rich diet and those on a chromium-deficient diet. Each group was fed a sugar solution to stimulate insulin. The rats fed the chromium-deficient diet secreted up to 50 percent less insulin during the study than did the rats on the chromium-rich diet. While rats and humans are considerably different, this study does suggest that chromium enhances the production of insulin as it is needed.
- *It tones out of shape muscles by increasing muscle mass.* Many health food shops sell chromium supplements as a muscle builder, but there's a catch—you have to exercise for the supplements to be effective. That's bad news for couch potatoes looking for a quick and easy fix.

- *It boosts longevity. All of the benefits just mentioned combine to add years to your life.* In studies on laboratory rats, those fed a diet rich in chromium picolinate lived one third longer than those that didn't receive the trace mineral. Researchers are unsure if chromium will help extend the human life span by a similar amount, but preliminary research is very promising.

There are no known dangers or side effects associated with chromium, and the FDA has not set a recommended daily allowance for the mineral. However, nutrition experts advise that you try to get as much chromium as you can from dietary sources because they tend to be more easily absorbed by the body.

Magnesium

Magnesium is an important mineral that shows great promise as an anti-aging facilitator. It plays a wide variety of roles within the body but is best known for promoting the absorption and use of other minerals, including calcium. Magnesium also helps move sodium and potassium across the cell membranes, aids in the metabolism of proteins, and activates a variety of important enzymes. What does this mean to you? It means strong bones and teeth, a healthy nervous system, a balanced metabolism, and well-functioning muscles—including the heart.

The importance of magnesium in maintaining youth can be seen in animals with magnesium deficiencies. In short, they age much faster than normal, are at higher risk of diabetes and heart attack, and show the classic signs of aging much earlier, including atherosclerosis, heartbeat irregularities, hypertension, and osteoporosis.

These problems have also been seen in people with low levels of magnesium. A Harvard University study found that people with a magnesium deficiency were more apt to have high blood pressure, a finding confirmed by a Swedish study that found that giving hypertension patients 360 milligrams of magnesium daily resulted in a dramatic—and potentially life-saving—reduction in blood pressure. And as far back as the 1950s, animal studies proved that high doses of magnesium can effectively reverse atherosclerotic plaques and improve blood flow to the heart.

There is also strong evidence that magnesium can facilitate glucose metabolism, lowering the risk of developing diabetes and making the condition easier to manage among those who already have it.

Are you getting adequate levels of magnesium? Probably not. Nutrition experts believe only one in four Americans is consuming sufficient levels of this vital mineral, and deficiencies are even higher among the elderly, who need it the most. The recommended daily allowance for magnesium is 350 milligrams for men eighteen and older and 300 milligrams for women eleven and older. However, many anti-aging experts believe even those levels are too low. Natural sources of magnesium include fish and seafood, fruits and fruit juice, green leafy vegetables, dairy products, nuts, and wheat germ. Magnesium is also available in supplement form.

When magnesium levels are low, cell membranes become less flexible and don't absorb calcium as well as they should. As a result, the integrity of the entire cell is placed in jeopardy. Magnesium also protects the mitochondria in the cells, which are necessary for energy production. When mitochondria are damaged in great numbers, researchers theorize, aging is accelerated. Consistently low magnesium levels make the problem worse by stimulating the production of inflammatory substances known as cytokines. These, in turn, create more free radicals and lead to even greater cell damage.

Magnesium is generally considered safe, though diarrhea may result when the mineral is consumed in high doses (700 milligrams daily over an extended period). In addition, people with a history of kidney disease or heart disease should consult their physician before taking magnesium supplements.

Selenium

Selenium was a little-considered mineral until the 1950s, when researchers first discovered its very important role in human health. Since then, numerous studies have placed it in the forefront of anti-aging research because of its suspected ability to prevent a variety of life-threatening conditions, including cancer and heart disease.

Selenium is important because it's an antioxidant, working with glutathione peroxidase to keep potentially damaging free radicals under control. It also plays a role in the metabolism of prostaglandins, important hormone-like compounds that affect several essential body functions. Natural sources of selenium include broccoli, cabbage, celery, cucumbers, garlic, onions, kidney, liver, chicken, whole-grain foods, seafood, and milk. It is also available in supplement form.

Selenium levels tend to drop precipitously as we age, which is why it's important that we maintain sufficient levels in our later years. In doing so, we can stay healthy and help ward off the effects of aging by preventing the formation of certain forms of cancer, reducing the risk of heart disease, and boosting immune function. Let's look at these benefits individually.

It's as a cancer-fighter that selenium really shines. Many studies have found that cancer rate is related to the amount of selenium we consume, with those who consume the lowest being most at risk. In Japan, for example, where people traditionally consume about 500 micrograms of selenium a day, the cancer rate is nearly five times lower than in countries where daily selenium intake is less. Cancer specialists have also found that the blood levels of selenium are lower in cancer patients than in healthy individuals.

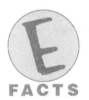

FACTS

Researchers are increasingly turning to birds as the subject of longevity and anti-aging studies because birds are biologically closer to humans than many other common tests subjects, such as worms or fruit flies.

Animal studies back up the importance of selenium in preventing cancer. In one telling experiment involving mice that were likely to get a specific form of cancer, only 10 percent of the rodents receiving selenium actually developed tumors, compared to 82 percent of the control group that did not receive the mineral.

Equally important is selenium's role in reducing heart disease and stroke, most likely by preventing blood platelets from sticking together and forming deadly clots. It also benefits the heart as an antioxidant, preventing the oxidation of LDL cholesterol.

Researchers have long suspected that selenium is instrumental to heart health, and a recent large-scale study in Finland finally confirmed it.

Researchers there found that subjects with the lowest levels of the mineral were three times more likely to die from heart disease than subjects with the highest levels. A separate study found that the lower a person's selenium level, the higher his or her potential degree of arterial blockage.

As an immunity booster, selenium can't be beat. Studies have shown that the mineral plays a vital role in keeping our immune system working as well at age sixty as at age twenty, and a deficiency can cause serious problems.

Of particular note is selenium's role as an antiviral agent. In one University of North Carolina study, researchers injected mice with a virus that usually is quite harmless. Then they artificially lowered the test animals' selenium levels. The result? The normally harmless virus suddenly became quite dangerous, breaking out of cells and attacking the muscles of the heart. This effect was not seen in a control group of infected mice who maintained healthy selenium levels.

Because of this remarkable antiviral action, some researchers speculate that selenium supplements may one day become part of the arsenal against AIDS and other life-threatening viral diseases. This makes sense because the HIV virus that causes AIDS is known to deplete the body's stores of selenium as part of its action.

Selenium, unlike many other common trace minerals, can be toxic in sustained daily doses of 700 to 1,000 micrograms, so doctors urge caution in its use as part of your anti-aging regimen. The Food and Drug Administration has not established a recommended daily allowance for selenium, though a daily dose between 50 and 200 micrograms is considered safe and effective. As a precaution, women should avoid taking high doses of selenium during pregnancy or while breastfeeding.

The Telomere Approach

Telomeres are lengths of DNA and protein that protect the tips of chromosomes in the nucleus of cells. These sections become a little bit shorter every time a cell divides, and when they eventually become too short, the cell dies or stops multiplying—a condition known as senescence. Some researchers theorize that senescence may act as a defense against cancer, which, as we know, is characterized by uncontrolled cell growth. That's good. However, biological aging may be a downside to telomere shrinkage. Based on this theory, a growing body of research now centers around extending telomere life and, thus, it's hoped, retarding the aging process.

Research into this area is still in the beginning stages. Scientists are still learning how telomeres function, and there is much debate over just how significant a role they play in the aging process. And even if it is proved that telomere shrinkage is the basis for organ deterioration, the questions remains, What can we do about it?

The role of telomeres can be seen in some of the most basic signs of aging, say researchers. Hair loss and skin wrinkling, for example, are caused by the inability of specific cells to multiply, presumably as a result of telomere shrinkage. Even more telling are certain human conditions that suggest a telomere defect, such as dyskeratosis congenita, or DKC. Individuals with this disorder have abnormally short telomeres and show early signs of aging, such as discolored skin, early-life anemia, and a weak immune system.

Laboratory studies in animals also suggest a strong link between shortened telomeres and signs of age. Mice that were genetically altered to have shortened telomeres demonstrated many of the classic signs of advanced physical decay at an abnormally young age. Their fur thinned and turned gray, their skin lost elasticity and became extremely thin, and they died long before they should have. They were also unable to reproduce, suggesting that the cells that should have become sperm and eggs simply couldn't survive.

The fact that these genetically altered mice didn't show all of the classic symptoms of aging, such as osteoporosis or other common age-related conditions, suggests that telomere shrinkage does not result in a traditional premature aging syndrome, note many researchers. However, it is believed to affect another aspect of the aging process—the inability to counteract chronic stress. And this, in turn, causes cells and systems to decay and age. This concept was bolstered by the fact that the mice with artificially shortened telomeres didn't heal nearly as well as unaltered mice of the same age when exposed to various stressors such as chemotherapy and minor surgery.

It must be noted that while animal studies help cast more light on the potential effects of telomere shrinkage, there is no proof that these results reflect similar action in human cells. Nonetheless, animal studies, as well as a better understanding of human telomere-defect conditions, are helping anti-aging researchers better understand the role of telomeres and possible ways to postpone or halt telomere shrinkage.

With dyskeratosis congenita, the cells that are most adversely affected are those that produce a telomere-restoring enzyme known as telomerase. This enzyme is found in the stem cells that eventually become eggs and sperm and in the cells used to rejuvenate the skin and blood. The obvious conclusion is that some cells need to turn on telomerase over the course of a normal lifespan in order to stay healthy and young.

The influence of telomerase as a possible youth preservative has not gone unnoticed. Some research firms are investigating the use of telomerase to maintain the ends of chromosomes and heal damaged or overworked organs in people of almost any age. In laboratory studies, the addition of the enzyme has noticeably increased the healthy lifespan of human eye, muscle, blood vessel, skin, and immune system cells.

Indeed, the potential benefits of telomerase supplementation are broad. If the enzyme proves effective in future research, it may one day be added to stem cells that generate new blood and skin cells as a way of allowing them to divide far longer and in turn alleviate some of the most common aspects of aging, such as slow healing of wounds and a flagging immune system.

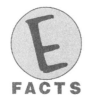

FACTS

The skin is considered an organ and weighs approximately 9 pounds if you're of average size.

The future may be closer than we think. Researchers recently reported tremendous success with a telomerase-based treatment that allowed cells to stay alive in culture and function normally when transplanted into a different animal. Such a procedure, advocates say, could one day reduce the risk of immune rejection in transplant patients, stimulate the creation of new blood vessels when arteries become clogged with plaque, prevent a wide variety of age-related diseases, and dramatically lengthen human longevity by helping organ cells continue to work far longer than they normally would.

The Genetic Approach

The year 2000 was a remarkable milestone in medical research with the announcement that researchers had finally completed a rough map of the human genome. The human genome is the array of nearly 80,000 genes that governs biological function and determines susceptibility to illnesses and, ultimately, how long we live.

The Human Genome Project was a huge undertaking more than a decade in the making and has tremendous implications for the prevention, diagnosis, and treatment of disease, as well as extending the human life span, say the researchers who participated in the project. "Mapping the human genome has been compared with putting a man on the moon but I believe it is more than that," said Dr. Michael Dexter, director of the Wellcome Trust, which helped fund, with the U.S. National Institutes of Health, the international Human Genome Project. "This is the outstanding achievement not only of our lifetime but perhaps in the history of mankind."

The genome sequence is comprised of more than 3 billion individual instructions, known as bases and represented by combinations of the letters A, C, G, and T. By decoding the sequences and looking for individual variations, researchers and doctors will one day be able to determine at an early age those likely to develop specific inherited diseases, eliminate many genetic disorders, and improve the treatment for those that cannot be eliminated. It is also hoped by anti-aging researchers that the eventual identification and cataloging of the genes responsible for aging will lead to gene therapy techniques that will dramatically extend the human life span well past its current accepted maximum of 120 years.

Many researchers predict that the benefits of the Human Genome Project will become available very quickly—possibly within the next ten years. Following is a quick look at what the coming decades may have to offer.

By 2010, the genome map is expected to identify people at the highest risk for specific genetic disorders, allowing doctors to monitor them earlier and treat them more effectively. An iron metabolism condition known as hemachromatosis is expected to become the model for this type of screening.

Within ten years, researchers say, genetic tests will be able to identify those at highest risk for lung cancer from smoking, and tests for colon cancer will limit colonoscopy screening to those who need it the most. In addition, a genetic test for prostate cancer could lead to more precise use of the prostate-specific antigen test by pinpointing men in whom the cancer is likely to progress the fastest. Genetic screening is also likely to determine risk for breast and ovarian cancer.

Genetic tests for a predisposition to coronary heart disease, diabetes, osteoporosis, and other conditions may help encourage susceptible individuals to begin preventive lifestyle changes before the diseases have a chance to develop. Early prevention and management could save countless lives, as well as billions of dollars in health care. Researchers also anticipate the wide availability of fetal screening, which will identify the presence of or probable risk for a wide variety of disorders, many of which can be treated in vitro or immediately after birth.

By 2020, doctors will likely rely on individual genetic variations in prescribing drugs and determining the most effective dose. In addition, pharmaceutical companies may begin re-examining drugs that were never marketed or taken off the market because of the risk of adverse reactions in the hope that they will benefit people with specific genetic conditions.

In addition, cancer specialists are expected to use drugs that precisely target a tumor's molecular "fingerprint." The drug Herceptin, which is marketed for the treatment of advanced breast cancer, is one such genetic-based designer compound.

The next twenty years may also see some amazing advances in the understanding, diagnosis, and treatment of mental illness as a result of the Human Genome Project. Of particular interest to researchers is the biological cause of debilitating mental illnesses such as schizophrenia and manic depression, as well as the possibility of a genetic test to gauge a person's susceptibility to such illnesses.

FACTS

Researchers at Oregon Health Sciences University in Portland have found a way to produce mice with genes that can be switched on and off, a development that could speed up the laboratory study of genes and their effect on disease.

By 2030, things should look brighter on the longevity front as researchers begin to identify the genes responsible for physical aging. By cataloging these genes and understanding better how they work, scientists say, we may be able to develop ways to influence them in a way that could slow or even postpone the aging process. The implications of such a find are astounding—if it can be done. And that, of course, remains the most important question.

The Real Bionic Man

Artificial organs have come a long way since 1982, when a sixty-one-year-old retired dentist named Barney Clark received the first Jarvik-7 artificial heart. The accompanying machinery that kept Clark alive was big and bulky, but it did the job, pumping blood through Clark's body for 112 days, until he finally succumbed to blood clots and other complications.

The Jarvik-7 is still used as an interim device, prolonging the life of heart patients until they can receive a transplant, but it quickly became evident that the machine was unfit for permanent service. It was too complicated, too unwieldy, and too inefficient for practical use, but it did open the door for a whole new generation of artificial organs, many of which, while still in the development stage, show tremendous promise in extending longevity.

In comparison to organs such as the liver and the pancreas, the heart is a relatively simple machine. It doesn't have to process chemicals, produce enzymes, or filter fluids—it just has to pump. Learning from the mistakes of earlier efforts, researchers working on the latest generation of artificial hearts have focused on miniaturization, the goal being a pump small enough for implantation without the bulky support system. And for the time being, they have also abandoned the idea of a whole mechanical heart, concentrating instead on devices that assist a failing heart until a suitable replacement can be found.

The most impressive example of heart-assist devices is the left ventricular assist device (LVAD). The device, which has been used for the past few years, is powered by a small battery pack worn outside the body. The battery pack is implanted in the abdomen and pumps blood that has been diverted from the left ventricle. The LVAD gives heart patients extra time to find a replacement organ.

The next step, say researchers, is a complete, implantable artificial heart without a bulky power system—a replacement organ that does the job just as well as the real thing. One of the fundamental concerns with an artificial heart is how it pumps blood. The old generation, characterized by the Jarvik-7, relied on a diaphragm system to move blood through the body. But scientists believe they have found a better, more reliable way—through the use of tiny, spinning impellers suspended within the device by magnets.

The McGowan Center has developed such a heart, an experimental organ known as the Streamliner. The small, lightweight device is implanted in the abdomen and pushes blood through the natural heart and arteries using a pair of tubes. Power comes from inductive coupling that transfers energy from a coil attached to a small battery worn on a belt to a second coil and battery implanted just beneath the skin. Such a system would allow the user almost total freedom—something Barney Clark never had. However, don't look for the Streamliner to become available anytime soon; it still requires many months of development before testing can begin, say its creators.

Making an artificial heart is child's play compared to manufacturing more complicated organs such as the liver, kidneys, or pancreas. Known as "smart" organs because of their complex function, mechanical replacements will almost certainly have to contain some organic tissue in order to work properly. The reason? Science is light years away from developing a mechanical version that can do the job even remotely as well as the real thing.

Most research into the creation of biochemical smart organs involves growing organ cells from humans or animals in culture, then placing the tissue in what is known as a bioreactor—a box or cylinder that keeps the tissue alive and functioning with a constant infusion of oxygen and necessary nutrients. In most systems currently under study, the bioreactor is placed in a larger machine through which blood is pumped via tubes. Implantable bioreactors are at least a decade away, say medical researchers, though temporary units that could be worn on the body may be a bit closer.

One of the most necessary artificial smart organs is the kidney. Currently, tens of thousands of Americans must undergo regular dialysis— an aggravating and time-consuming procedure—just to stay alive. And dialysis isn't perfect. Healthy kidneys filter urea waste products from the blood, and the organs' tubules reclaim and send back into the body important nutrients such as sugars and salts acquired from the filtrate. Unfortunately, today's dialysis machines simply can't accomplish the second task.

The answer, say researchers, is a bioartificial kidney that would combine specially engineered tissue with some kind of mechanical housing. An artificial organ of this type would be able to handle all of the functions of a real kidney, making traditional dialysis obsolete for most people.

Such an organ is currently under study at the University of Michigan. Researchers there have cultured proximal tubule cells from pig kidneys and enmeshed them along extremely thin fibers inside a small filtration cartridge. The cartridge is contained in a larger machine, which filters the patient's blood and returns needed nutrients that otherwise would be lost. The system has been tested successfully on dogs and, as of this writing, is awaiting FDA approval for testing on humans.

The University of Michigan bioartificial kidney will most likely be used as a temporary fix for people in acute kidney failure, a lifesaving stop-gap measure until a transplant kidney can be found. However, its creators believe that it's only a matter of time before a smaller, wearable version is perfected. Such a device, while certainly not as ideal as a real kidney, could reduce dialysis time by as much as 50 percent and perhaps even eliminate it completely.

Even more complicated than an artificial kidney is a man-made pancreas. However, the effort is well worth it, say advocates, because such a device could dramatically improve the health and quality of life for millions of people with insulin-dependent diabetes.

People with insulin-dependent diabetes must regularly check their blood sugar and inject themselves with insulin to keep the condition under control. One of the biggest drawbacks to this very common approach, however, is that there is no absolute way of knowing exactly how much insulin is needed. In most cases, patients are left to make an educated guess. The resulting fluctuations in glucose levels over many years are believed to be the cause of the most common complications associated with diabetes, including heart disease and vision problems.

The ideal artificial pancreas would take the guessing out of glucose control by "listening" to feedback from the body in determining exactly how much insulin to release and when to do it. Currently in the development stage is the PancreAssist from Circe Biomedical in Lexington, Massachusetts. This system monitors the body's chemistry to determine how much insulin is needed, then releases it at just the right time.

The PancreAssist is a plastic-cased, implantable tubular membrane surrounded by insulin-producing pig islets. As the user's blood flows through the center of the tube, the islets monitor his or her glucose levels and produce insulin, which is diffused through the membrane into the user's bloodstream as needed. The membrane also plays an important role in protecting the pig islets from the body's natural defense systems, which would render them useless if given the chance. If all goes well, clinical testing on humans could begin within the next couple of years, say officials with Circe Biomedical.

An equally important but even more complex organ is the liver. Located in the upper right region of the abdomen, it plays an important role in the utilization of absorbed foods, including the conversion of excess glucose into glycogen, which it stores and reconverts into glucose when required. The liver also breaks down excess amino acids into urea and stores and metabolizes fat, among other duties. When the liver becomes damaged from disease (hepatitis C) or abuse (alcoholism), it can't function as well as it should. Liver failure usually means death.

The liver is a transplantable organ, but the number of recipients far exceeds the number of donor organs, hence the need for an artificial assist. A functioning artificial liver that could last a lifetime would be a godsend to innumerable patients who wait helplessly while their livers fail, but such a machine is many, many years away. A better, more manageable option is a bioartificial system that could take over much of the function of the liver for a short period, just long enough for the ailing organ to regenerate and repair itself. Some experts believe that even a week's respite would be sufficient to allow many damaged livers to fix themselves sufficiently to return to near-normal function.

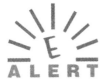

The completion of the human genome map is the first step toward unprecedented breakthroughs in medical research. In the not too distant future, almost everyone will be able to determine through a simple blood or saliva test whether he or she is predisposed to a wide variety of medical disorders. But what of the risks that come from that knowledge? What kinds of protection will we need to keep private companies and government agencies from using this information against us? Former President Clinton and individuals involved with the Human Genome Project have urged Congress to pass a pending bill that would prohibit discrimination—including insurance denial—based on genetic information.

Not surprisingly, several companies are hard at work developing such as system, including Circe Biomedical, which created the experimental HepatAssist system in collaboration with liver specialists at Cedars-Sinai Medical Center in Los Angeles. The HepatAssist uses pig liver cells to eliminate toxins from the blood, much like prototypical bioartificial kidneys do, say researchers. A plastic cartridge lined with engineered cells fits in a larger machine though which blood is passed for cleaning. Ideally, patients will use the machine approximately six hours a day for a week—sufficient time, it's hoped, for the liver to adequately repair itself.

Bioartificial organs are just one approach researchers are examining in their quest to extend the lives of people whose bodies are failing for whatever reason. Another approach, more science fiction than fact at this point, but still worth discussing, is a concept known as xenotransplantation, in which specially engineered organs derived from other species are transplanted into ailing humans. Rejection of the new organs could be prevented, say researchers, by placing imbuing human genes into the organs, which would then be engineered not to stimulate the body's natural immune defenses.

The Man-Made Body

In the camp TV series *The Six Million Dollar Man*, Col. Steve Austin (Lee Majors) is "made better" when fitted with atomic-powered body parts after being severely injured while testing a moon-landing craft. When Austin recovers, he finds that government doctors have given him mechanical legs that allow him to run extremely fast, a super-strong right arm, and an artificial left eye capable of extraordinary vision.

Of course, *The Six Million Dollar Man* is pure science fiction, but the astounding advances mentioned in the show are closer than you may assume. We already have prosthetic limbs, including artificial arms and hands that can grasp (although, admittedly, such organs are nowhere near as strong as those given Col. Austin), and a wide array of artificial joints. In addition, mechanical larynxes allow the voiceless to speak and state-of-the-art cochlear implants give the gift of hearing to those who never had it before. And, in the not too distant future, an astounding collaboration of computer and brain may mean sight for millions of people who otherwise would be totally blind.

We have, indeed, come a long way from the days when metal hooks were the only substitute for missing hands. Ongoing advances in computer science, biotechnical science, and prosthetic technology have made almost anything possible in the realm of organ and system replacement—which is good news for the people of today and great news for the people of tomorrow. If technology continues at its current pace, say futurists, the loss of almost any organ will be a minor inconvenience at best. If a replacement can't be grown in a laboratory from the patient's own stem cells, then it will be manufactured.

Carried to extremes, the easy replacement of damaged or failing body parts could usher in an era of hyperlongevity; people will visit their doctors for a quick "organ fix" much like they visit their mechanics when a car part needs replacing. It's just science fiction now, but you never know what tomorrow will bring.

What the Future Holds

As with nearly everything connected with scientific research, we've only seen the tip of the iceberg when it comes to anti-aging research. In years and decades to come, concepts and ideas so far fetched as to be outside the realm of current thought will almost certainly prove to be tomorrow's advances, adding yet more years to the ever-lengthening human life span.

Our risk of diseases both common and obscure will be determined while we're in the womb, and that risk will be easily and inexpensively eliminated through state-of-the-art gene therapy. The ailments that we do develop over our lifetime, many of which cut short the lives of our ancestors, will be cured through nanotechnology. Can you imagine millions of microscopic robots living within our bodies, repairing cell damage, keeping our immune system strong, looking for and destroying disease-causing pathogens?

Hearts, livers, and kidneys worn out with age will be replaced with organs cloned from our own uniquely engineered stem cells or acquired from transgenic animals whose DNA has been altered so that their tissue won't be rejected by our sensitive immune defenses. Limbs rendered useless by illness or accidents will be replaced with electronic arms and legs that look and work just like the real thing. Computer chips will be implanted in our brains to constantly monitor our health and well-being and let us know when problems are imminent.

The future is a vast universe of unknown ideas and unexplored possibilities. We probably won't be around long enough to see most of the advances already noted, but they will surely benefit our children and grandchildren. If science maintains its current pace, the "Immortal Man" will be here sooner than we think

Appendix: Organizations and Associations

Health

✉ **Administration on Aging**
330 Independence Avenue SW
Washington, DC 20201
Tel: 202-619-0724

✉ **Aging Network Services**
4400 East-West Highway
Bethesda, MD 20814
Tel: 301-657-4329

✉ **Alzheimer's Association**
919 North Michigan
Chicago, IL 60611
Tel: 800-272-3900

✉ **American Academy of Dermatology**
930 North Meacham Road
P.O. Box 4014
Schaumberg, IL 60168-4014
Tel: 847-330-0230

✉ **American Academy of Ophthalmology**
P.O. Box 7424
San Francisco, CA 94120-7424
Tel: 800-684-9788
In San Francisco, call 415-561-8500

✉ **American Association of Cardiovascular and Pulmonary Rehabilitation**
7611 Elmwood Avenue, Suite 201
Middleton, WI 53562
Tel: 608-831-6989

✉ **American Association of Retired Persons (AARP)**
601 E Street NW
Washington, DC 20049
Tel: 202-434-2277

✉ **American Cancer Society, Inc.**
National Headquarters
1599 Clifton Road NE
Atlanta, GA 30329-4251
Tel: 404-320-3333
For the number of your local
Cancer Society, call 800-227-2345

✉ **American College of Sports Medicine**
P.O. Box 1440
Indianapolis, IN 46206
Tel: 317-637-9200

✉ **American Diabetes Association**
1660 Duke Street
Alexandria, VA 22314
Tel: 800-DIABETES (342-2383)

✉ **American Dietetic Association**
216 West Jackson Boulevard, Suite 800
Chicago, IL 60606
Tel: 800-366-1655 (Nutrition Hotline)

✉ **American Psychological Association**
750 First Street NE
Washington, DC 20002
Tel: 202-336-5500

✉ **American Sleep Disorders Association**
1610 14th Street NW
Rochester, MN 55901
Tel: 507-287-6006

✉ **American Society of Plastic Surgeons**
444 East Algonquin Road
Arlington Heights, IL 60005
Tel: 888-475-2742

✉ **Anxiety Disorders Association of America**
Dept. B, P.O. Box 96505
Washington, DC 20077-7140
Tel: 301-231-9350

✉ **Arthritis Foundation**
1314 Spring Street
Atlanta, GA 30309
P.O. Box 19000
Atlanta, GA 30326
Tel: 800-283-7800
In Atlanta: 404-872-7100

✉ **American Heart Association**
7272 Greenville Avenue
Dallas, TX 75231-4596
Tel: 214-373-6300
For the number of your local Heart
Association, call 800-AHA-USA1 (242-8721)

✉ **American Institute for Cancer Research**
1759 R Street NW
Washington, DC 20009
Tel: 800-843-8114

✉ **Center for Mind/Body Medicine**
5225 Connecticut Avenue NW, Suite 414
Washington, DC 20015
Tel: 202-966-7338

✉ **Council for Responsible Nutrition**
1300 19th Street NW, Suite 310
Washington, DC 20036
Tel: 202-872-1488

✉ **Depression After Delivery**
P.O. Box 1282
Morrisville, PA 19067
Tel: 908-575-9121

✉ **Dietary Guidelines for Americans**
Consumer Information Center
Pueblo, CO 81009
Free with self-addressed, stamped envelope

✉ **Environmental Protection Agency**
Washington, DC
Public Information Center: 202-260-2080
Safe Drinking Water Hot Line: 800-426-4791

✉ **Food and Drug Administration**
5600 Fishers Lane
Rockville, MD 20857-0001
Tel: 888-463-6332

✉ **International Academy of Alternative Health and Medicine**
218 Avenue B
Redondo Beach, CA 90277
Tel: 310-540-0564

✉ **International Federation on Aging**
601 E Street NW
Washington, DC 20049
Tel: 202-434-2427

✉ **National Association of Area Agencies on Aging**
11112 16th Street NW
Washington, DC 20036
Tel: 202-296-8130

✉ **National Council on Aging**
409 Third Street SW, Suite 200
Washington, DC 20024
Tel: 800-424-9046
In DC: 202-479-1200

✉ **National Eye Institute**
Information Office, Building 31,
Room 6A32
31 Center Drive MSC 2510
Bethesda, MD 20892-2510
Tel: 301-496-5248

✉ **National Health Information Center**
P.O. Box 1133
Washington, DC 20013
Tel: 301-565-4167

✉ **National Heart, Lung, and Blood Institute Information Center**
P.O. Box 30105
Bethesda, MD 20824-0105
Tel: 301-251-1222

✉ **National Hypertension Association**
324 East 30th Street
New York, NY 10016
Tel: 212-889-3557

✉ **National Institute on Aging's Alzheimer's Disease Education and Referral Center**
P.O. Box 8250
Silver Spring, MD 20907-8250
Tel: 800-438-4380

✉ **National Institutes of Health**
National Institute on Aging
Information Center
P.O. Box 8057
Gaithersburg, MD 20898-8057
Tel: 800-222-2225 (Publication Info)
or 301-496-1752 (Information Center)

✉ **National Institute of Mental Health**
5600 Fishers Lane, Room 7C-02
Rockville, MD 20857
Tel: 301-443-4513

✉ **National Institute of Neurological Disorders and Stroke**
31 Center Drive, MSC 2540
Bethesda, MD 20892-2540
Tel: 800-352-9424

⊠ **National Kidney and Urologic Diseases Information Clearinghouse**
3 Information Way
Bethesda, MD 20892-3560
Tel: 301-654-4415

⊠ **National Osteoporosis Foundation**
1150 17th Street NW, Suite 500
Washington, DC 20036-4603
Tel: 202-223-2226

⊠ **National Parkinson Foundation**
1501 NW 9th Avenue
Miami, FL 33136
Tel: 800-327-4545

⊠ **National Women's Health Information Center**
Tel: 800-994-9662

⊠ **National Women's Health Network**
514 10th Street NW, Suite 400
Washington, DC 20004
Tel: 202-347-1140

⊠ **North American Menopause Society**
P.O. Box 94527
Cleveland, OH 44101-4527
Tel: 440-442-7550

⊠ **Older Women's League (OWL)**
666 11th Street NW, Suite 700
Washington, DC 20001
Tel: 202-783-6686

⊠ **Osteoporosis and Related Bone Diseases National Resource Center**
1150 17th Street NW, Suite 500
Washington, DC 20036-4603
Tel: 800-624-BONE (2663)
In DC, call 202-223-0344

⊠ **President's Council on Physical Fitness and Sports**
200 Independence Avenue SW, Room 738-H
Washington DC 20201
Tel: 202-690-9000

⊠ **Skin Cancer Foundation**
245 Fifth Avenue, Suite 1403 NW
New York, NY 10016
Tel: 800-SKIN-490 (754-6490)
In New York, call 212-725-5176

Aging Research

⊠ **Academy of Pharmaceutical Research and Science**
2215 Constitution Avenue NW
Washington, DC 20037
Tel: 202-628-4410

⊠ **Aeron Lifecycles**
1933 Davis Street, Suite 310
San Leandro, CA 94577
Tel: 800-631-7900

✉ **Alcor Life Extension Foundation**
7895 East Acoma Drive, Suite 110
Scottsdale, AZ 85260-6916
Tel: 877-462-5267

✉ **Alliance for Aging Research**
2021 K Street NW, Suite 304
Washington, DC 20006
Tel: 202-293-2856

✉ **American Academy of Anti-aging Medicine**
1341 West Fullerton Avenue, Suite 111
Chicago, IL 60614
Tel: 773-528-1000

✉ **American Federation for Aging Research**
1414 Avenue of the Americas, 18th Floor
New York, NY 10019
Tel: 212-752-2327

✉ **American Geriatrics Society, Inc.**
770 Lexington Avenue, Suite 300
New York, NY 10021
Tel: 212-308-1414

✉ **American Society of Human Genetics**
9650 Rockville Pike
Bethesda, MD 20814
Tel: 301-571-1825

✉ **Bio Research Institute**
4492 Camino de la Plaza, Suite TIJ-1063
San Diego, CA 92173-3097
Tel: 800-291-1508

✉ **Dana Alliance for Brain Initiatives**
745 Fifth Avenue, Suite 700
New York, NY 10151
Tel: 212-223-4040

✉ **Division on Aging**
Harvard Medical School
643 Huntington Avenue
Boston, MA 02115
Tel: 617-432-1840

✉ **Harvard Health Letter**
154 Longwood Avenue
Boston, MA 02115
Tel: 617-432-1485

✉ **Health & Longevity Newsletter**
105 West Monument Street
Baltimore, MD 21201
Tel: 410-223-2611

✉ **Journal of Longevity Research**
330 Washington Boulevard, Suite 900
Marina del Rey, CA 90290
Tel: 310-577-8416

✉ **Life Extension Foundation**
P.O. Box 229120
Hollywood, CA 33022
Tel: 800-841-5433

✉ **National Foundation for Brain Research**
1250 24th Street NW, Suite 300
Washington, DC 20037
Tel: 202-293-5453

Books

- *Age-Proof Your Body: Your Complete Guide to Lifelong Vitality,* by Elizabeth Somer, M.A., R.D. (Quill)

- *Age Right: Turn Back the Clock with a Proven Personalized Antiaging Program,* by Karlis Ullis, M.D., with Greg Ptacek (Simon & Schuster)

- *The Anti-aging Plan: Strategies and Recipes for Extending Your Healthy Years,* by Roy L. Walford and Lisa Walford (Four Walls Eight Windows)

- *Beyond the 120 Year Diet: How to Double Your Vital Years,* by Roy L. Walford (Four Walls Eight Windows)

- *Brain Longevity,* by Dharma Singh Khalsa, M.D., with Cameron Stauth (Warner Books)

- *Dare to Be 100,* by Walter M. Bortz II, M.D. (Fireside)

- *Earl Mindell's Anti-aging Bible,* by Earl Mindell, R.Ph., Ph.D. (Fireside)

- *Gary Null's Ultimate Anti-aging Program,* by Gary Null, Ph.D. (Kensington)

- *Live Now, Age Later: Proven Ways to Slow Down the Clock,* by Isadore Rosenfeld, M.D. (Warner Books)

- *Living to 100: Lessons in Living to Your Maximum Potential at Any Age,* by Thomas T. Perls, M.D., M.P.H., and Margery Hutter Silver, Ed.D., with John F. Lauerman (Basic Books)

- *One Hundred and Twenty Year Diet: How to Double Your Vital Years,* by Roy L. Walford (Simon & Schuster)

- *Prescription for Long Life: Essential Remedies for Longevity,* by Dr. Mitchell Kurk and Dr. Morton Walker (Avery)

- *RealAge: Are You As Young As You Can Be?,* by Michael F. Roizen, M.D. (Cliff Street Books)

- *Retardation of Aging and Disease by Dietary Restriction,* by Richard Weindruch and Roy L. Walford (Charles C. Thomas)

- *Staying Healthy in a Risky Environment: The New York University Medical Center Family Guide,* Arthur C. Upton, M.D., Medical Editor; Eden Graber, M.S., Editor (Simon & Schuster)

- *Stop Aging Now!: The Ultimate Plan for Staying Young and Reversing the Aging Process,* by Jean Carper (HarperPerennial)

- *Stopping the Clock: Dramatic Breakthroughs in Anti-aging and Age Reversal Techniques,* by Dr. Ronald Klatz and Dr. Robert Goldman (Bantam Books)

- *Successful Aging,* by John W. Rowe, M.D., and Robert L. Kahn, Ph.D. (Dell)

Web Sites

Putting the words *anti-aging* and *longevity* into your computer's search engine will immediately introduce you to hundreds of Web sites devoted to anti-aging, longevity, and associated products and services. A growing number of these sites sell drugs, hormones, herbs, and other anti-aging compounds, many of which have not been approved by the Food and Drug Administration or thoroughly tested for safety and efficacy—so be very cautious. Following is a small selection of information-based health and anti-aging Web sites:

Ageless Design
(offers informative monthly newsletter for Alzheimer's patients and caregivers)
www.agelessdesign.com

American Academy of Anti-aging Medicine
www.worldhealth.net

Anti-aging Lifestyle, Anti-aging Therapy, Anti-aging Medicine, Anti-aging Science
www.anti-age.com

International Academy of Alternative and Anti-aging Medicine
www.gvi.com/givweb/iaam

International Federation on Aging
www.ifa-fiv.org

The Life Extension Foundation
www.lef.org

Northwestern Mutual: The Longevity Game (simple online game that determines how long you'll live based on lifestyle, medical history, and family history)
www.northwesternmutual.com

Rejuvenation & Longevity Foundation
www.anti-aging.org

Rx for Wellness
www.rxforwellness.com

Index

Magnetic resonance imaging (MRI), 38
Majors, Lee, 272
Mammogram, 10, 11
Managed health care, 5–7
Marriage, role of, 197–98
Massages, 102–3
Masters and Johnson, 108
McGowan Center, 268
McKay, Clive M., 248
Measles vaccine, 102
Medical breakthroughs, 30. *See also* Research
Medical Center of Georgia, 104
Medical College of Wisconsin, 250
Meditation, 103–4
Melanoma, 110
Melatonin, 254–57
Memorization, 40–41
Memory, 29, 38–40
Memory loss, 130, 131, 133. *See also* Alzheimer's disease; Dementia
Men
  anti-aging and, 219–22
  exercise and, 220–21
  exercise tips, 52–53
  lifestyle and, 221–22
  nutrition and, 219–20
Menopause, 19, 28
  osteoporosis and, 121, 147–48
Mental acuity. *See also* Brain
  maintaining, 33, 39–42
  myths on, 13
  nutrition and, 72–75

social support systems and, 211–13
stimulation of, 14, 26, 33, 35–42
Mercury, 162, 184, 188–89
Metabolism
  aging and, 20, 24, 45, 124
  magnesium and, 259–60
Metals, toxicity of, 162–63
Methionine, 73
Microorganisms, 160
Milwaukee VA Medical Center, 250
Minerals
  anti-aging and, 257–62
  benefits of, 65–68
  mental acuity and, 74–75
Moderation, 48
Moisturizers, 14
Monoterpenes, 61
Monounsaturated fats, 71
Morphine, 78
Mumps vaccine, 102
Muscle injury, 182
Muscle tone
  changes in, 24
  strengthening, 45–46
Myeloma, 119
Myocarditis, 139–40
Myths on aging, 13–15

N

National Cancer Institute, 70, 119
National Center for Health Statistics, 179
National Council on Alcoholism and Drug Dependence, 208

National Heart, Lung, and Blood Institute, 230
National Institute on Aging, 18, 30
National Institutes of Health, 251, 265
National Safe Workplace Institute, 181
National Safety Council, 181
Negative attitude, 31–32
Nerve-cell loss, 189
Nervous system damage, 189
Neuroendocrine Theory, 19
Night blindness, 26
Nitrates, 163–64
Nitroglycerin, 138
Noise, in the workplace, 182, 185
Non-insulin-dependent diabetes, 122–23, 153
Nonionizing radiation, 185–86
Nucleic acids, 23
Nutrition, 12
  benefits of, 44–45, 57–76, 94
  children and, 229–30
  men and, 219–20
  mental acuity and, 72–75
  role of, 57–58
  women and, 224–26

O

Obesity, 49, 63
  preventing, 151
Occupational hazards, 180–88
  biological, 186–87
  chemical, 183–84

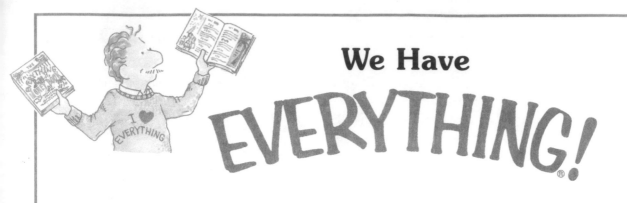

We Have EVERYTHING!

Everything® **After College Book**
$12.95, 1-55850-847-3

Everything® **American History Book**
$12.95, 1-58062-531-2

Everything® **Angels Book**
$12.95, 1-58062-398-0

Everything® **Anti-Aging Book**
$12.95, 1-58062-565-7

Everything® **Astrology Book**
$12.95, 1-58062-062-0

Everything® **Baby Names Book**
$12.95, 1-55850-655-1

Everything® **Baby Shower Book**
$12.95, 1-58062-305-0

Everything® **Baby's First Food Book**
$12.95, 1-58062-512-6

Everything® **Baby's First Year Book**
$12.95, 1-58062-581-9

Everything® **Barbeque Cookbook**
$12.95, 1-58062-316-6

Everything® **Bartender's Book**
$9.95, 1-55850-536-9

Everything® **Bedtime Story Book**
$12.95, 1-58062-147-3

Everything® **Bicycle Book**
$12.00, 1-55850-706-X

Everything® **Build Your Own Home Page**
$12.95, 1-58062-339-5

Everything® **Business Planning Book**
$12.95, 1-58062-491-X

Everything® **Casino Gambling Book**
$12.95, 1-55850-762-0

Everything® **Cat Book**
$12.95, 1-55850-710-8

Everything® **Chocolate Cookbook**
$12.95, 1-58062-405-7

Everything® **Christmas Book**
$15.00, 1-55850-697-7

Everything® **Civil War Book**
$12.95, 1-58062-366-2

Everything® **College Survival Book**
$12.95, 1-55850-720-5

Everything® **Computer Book**
$12.95, 1-58062-401-4

Everything® **Cookbook**
$14.95, 1-58062-400-6

Everything® **Cover Letter Book**
$12.95, 1-58062-312-3

Everything® **Crossword and Puzzle Book**
$12.95, 1-55850-764-7

Everything® **Dating Book**
$12.95, 1-58062-185-6

Everything® **Dessert Book**
$12.95, 1-55850-717-5

Everything® **Digital Photography Book**
$12.95, 1-58062-574-6

Everything® **Dog Book**
$12.95, 1-58062-144-9

Everything® **Dreams Book**
$12.95, 1-55850-806-6

Everything® **Etiquette Book**
$12.95, 1-55850-807-4

Everything® **Fairy Tales Book**
$12.95, 1-58062-546-0

Everything® **Family Tree Book**
$12.95, 1-55850-763-9

Everything® **Fly-Fishing Book**
$12.95, 1-58062-148-1

Everything® **Games Book**
$12.95, 1-55850-643-8

Everything® **Get-A-Job Book**
$12.95, 1-58062-223-2

Everything® **Get Published Book**
$12.95, 1-58062-315-8

Everything® **Get Ready for Baby Book**
$12.95, 1-55850-844-9

Everything® **Ghost Book**
$12.95, 1-58062-533-9

Everything® **Golf Book**
$12.95, 1-55850-814-7

Everything® **Grammar and Style Book**
$12.95, 1-58062-573-8

Everything® **Guide to Las Vegas**
$12.95, 1-58062-438-3

Everything® **Guide to New York City**
$12.95, 1-58062-314-X

Everything® **Guide to Walt Disney World®, Universal Studios®, and Greater Orlando, 2nd Edition**
$12.95, 1-58062-404-9

Everything® **Guide to Washington, D.C.**
$12.95, 1-58062-313-1

Everything® **Guitar Book**
$12.95, 1-58062-555-X

Everything® **Herbal Remedies Book**
$12.95, 1-58062-331-X

Everything® **Home-Based Business Book**
$12.95, 1-58062-364-6

Everything® **Homebuying Book**
$12.95, 1-58062-074-4

Everything® **Homeselling Book**
$12.95, 1-58062-304-2

Available wherever books are sold!
Visit us at everything.com

Everything® **Home Improvement Book**
$12.95, 1-55850-718-3

Everything® **Horse Book**
$12.95, 1-58062-564-9

Everything® **Hot Careers Book**
$12.95, 1-58062-486-3

Everything® **Internet Book**
$12.95, 1-58062-073-6

Everything® **Investing Book**
$12.95, 1-58062-149-X

Everything® **Jewish Wedding Book**
$12.95, 1-55850-801-5

Everything® **Job Interviews Book**
$12.95, 1-58062-493-6

Everything® **Lawn Care Book**
$12.95, 1-58062-487-1

Everything® **Leadership Book**
$12.95, 1-58062-513-4

Everything® **Learning Spanish Book**
$12.95, 1-58062-575-4

Everything® **Low-Fat High-Flavor Cookbook**
$12.95, 1-55850-802-3

Everything® **Magic Book**
$12.95, 1-58062-418-9

Everything® **Managing People Book**
$12.95, 1-58062-577-0

Everything® **Microsoft® Word 2000 Book**
$12.95, 1-58062-306-9

Everything® **Money Book**
$12.95, 1-58062-145-7

Everything® **Mother Goose Book**
$12.95, 1-58062-490-1

Everything® **Mutual Funds Book**
$12.95, 1-58062-419-7

Everything® **One-Pot Cookbook**
$12.95, 1-58062-186-4

Everything® **Online Business Book**
$12.95, 1-58062-320-4

Everything® **Online Genealogy Book**
$12.95, 1-58062-402-2

Everything® **Online Investing Book**
$12.95, 1-58062-338-7

Everything® **Online Job Search Book**
$12.95, 1-58062-365-4

Everything® **Pasta Book**
$12.95, 1-55850-719-1

Everything® **Pregnancy Book**
$12.95, 1-58062-146-5

Everything® **Pregnancy Organizer**
$15.00, 1-58062-336-0

Everything® **Project Management Book**
$12.95, 1-58062-583-5

Everything® **Puppy Book**
$12.95, 1-58062-576-2

Everything® **Quick Meals Cookbook**
$12.95, 1-58062-488-X

Everything® **Resume Book**
$12.95, 1-58062-311-5

Everything® **Romance Book**
$12.95, 1-58062-566-5

Everything® **Sailing Book**
$12.95, 1-58062-187-2

Everything® **Saints Book**
$12.95, 1-58062-534-7

Everything® **Selling Book**
$12.95, 1-58062-319-0

Everything® **Spells and Charms Book**
$12.95, 1-58062-532-0

Everything® **Stress Management Book**
$12.95, 1-58062-578-9

Everything® **Study Book**
$12.95, 1-55850-615-2

Everything® **Tall Tales, Legends, and Outrageous Lies Book**
$12.95, 1-58062-514-2

Everything® **Tarot Book**
$12.95, 1-58062-191-0

Everything® **Time Management Book**
$12.95, 1-58062-492-8

Everything® **Toasts Book**
$12.95, 1-58062-189-9

Everything® **Total Fitness Book**
$12.95, 1-58062-318-2

Everything® **Trivia Book**
$12.95, 1-58062-143-0

Everything® **Tropical Fish Book**
$12.95, 1-58062-343-3

Everything® **Vitamins, Minerals, and Nutritional Supplements Book**
$12.95, 1-58062-496-0

Everything® **Wedding Book, 2nd Edition**
$12.95, 1-58062-190-2

Everything® **Wedding Checklist**
$7.95, 1-58062-456-1

Everything® **Wedding Etiquette Book**
$7.95, 1-58062-454-5

Everything® **Wedding Organizer**
$15.00, 1-55850-828-7

Everything® **Wedding Shower Book**
$7.95, 1-58062-188-0

Everything® **Wedding Vows Book**
$7.95, 1-58062-455-3

Everything® **Wine Book**
$12.95, 1-55850-808-2

Everything® **World War II Book**
$12.95, 1-58062-572-X

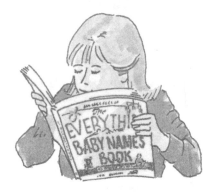

Everything® is a registered trademark of Adams Media Corporation.

We Have

EVERYTHING KIDS'®!

Everything® Kids' Baseball Book
$9.95, 1-58062-489-8

Everything® Kids' Online Book
$9.95, 1-58062-394-8

Everything® Kids' Joke Book
$9.95, 1-58062-495-2

Everything® Kids' Puzzle Book
$9.95, 1-58062-323-9

Everything® Kids' Mazes Book
$6.95, 1-58062-558-4

Everything® Kids' Science Experiments Book
$6.95, 1-58062-557-6

Everything® Kids' Money Book
$9.95, 1-58062-322-0

Everything® Kids' Space Book
$9.95, 1-58062-395-6

Everything® Kids' Nature Book
$9.95, 1-58062-321-2

Everything® Kids' Witches and Wizards Book
$9.95, 1-58062-396-4

Available wherever books are sold!

For more information, or to order,
call 800-872-5627 or visit everything.com

Adams Media Corporation, 57 Littlefield Street, Avon, MA 02322

Everything® is a registered trademark of Adams Media Corporation.